Dx/Rx:

Lung Cancer

Second Edition

Christopher G. Azzoli, MD
Memorial Sloan-Kettering Cancer Center
Department of Medicine
Thoracic Oncology Service
New York, New York

Series Editor: Manish A. Shah, MD
Director of Gastrointestinal Oncology
Weill Cornell Medical College/New York–Presbyterian
Hospital
New York, New York

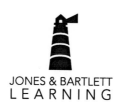

JONES & BARTLETT
LEARNING

World Headquarters
Jones & Bartlett Learning
5 Wall Street
Burlington, MA 01803
978-443-5000
info@jblearning.com
www.jblearning.com

Jones & Bartlett Learning books and products are available through most bookstores and online booksellers. To contact Jones & Bartlett Learning directly, call 800-832-0034, fax 978-443-8000, or visit our website, www.jblearning.com.

Substantial discounts on bulk quantities of Jones & Bartlett Learning publications are available to corporations, professional associations, and other qualified organizations. For details and specific discount information, contact the special sales department at Jones & Bartlett Learning via the above contact information or send an email to specialsales@jblearning.com.

Production Credits
Executive Publisher: Christopher Davis
Associate Editor: Laura Burns
Production Assistant: Sarah Burke
Marketing Manager: Rebecca Rockel
Manufacturing and Inventory Control Supervisor: Amy Bacus
Composition: Westchester Book Group
Cover Design: Kate Ternullo/Kristin E. Parker
Cover Image: © Sebastian Kaulitzki/ShutterStock, Inc.
Printing and Binding: Edwards Brothers Malloy
Cover Printing: Edwards Brothers Malloy

Library of Congress Cataloging-in-Publication Data
Azzoli, Christopher G.
  Dx/Rx. Lung cancer / Christopher G. Azzoli.—2nd ed.
    p. ; cm.
  Lung cancer
  Includes bibliographical references and index.
  ISBN-13: 978-1-4496-0039-6
  ISBN-10: 1-4496-0039-5
  I. Title. II. Title: Lung cancer.
  [DNLM: 1. Lung Neoplasms—Handbooks. WF 39]
  616.99'424—dc23
                                    2011043971
6048

Printed in the United States of America
16 15 14 13 12   10 9 8 7 6 5 4 3 2 1

Other books in the Dx/Rx Oncolo Jones & Bartlett Learning

Dx/Rx: Breast Cancer, Second Edition
Diana E. Lake

Dx/Rx: Cervical Cancer: Diagnosis and Treatment of Pre-cancerous Lesions (CIN) and Cervical Cancer, Second Edition
Katina Robison and Don S. Dizon

Dx/Rx: Colorectal Cancer
Hole· and Ki Yo

Dx/Rx: Genitourinary Oncology: Cancer of the Kidney, Bladder, and Testis, Second Edition
Matthew D. Galsky

Dx/Rx: Gynecologic Cancer
Don S. Dizon and Susana M. Campos

Dx/Rx: Head and Neck Cancer
Kenneth S. Hu, Robert I. Haddad, and Adam Jacobson

Dx/Rx: Leukemia, Second Edition
John M. Burke

Dx/Rx: Lymphoma, Second Edition
Daniel O. Persky

Dx/Rx: Melanoma
Richard D. Carvajal

Dx/Rx: Palliative Cancer Care
V. Tim Malhotra and Natalie Moryl

Dx/Rx: Pancreatic Cancer
Maeve Lowery and Eileen M. O'Reilly

Dx/Rx: Prostate Cancer, Second Edition
Lewis J. Kampel

Dx/Rx: Upper Gastrointestinal Malignancies: Cancers of the Stomach and Esophagus
Manish A. Shah

Dedication

To my wife, Lisa. Thank you for giving me the time and freedom to work at something that I love, and for giving me four wonderful daughters, Maxine, Isabelle, Francesca, and Lily.

Contents

Editor's Preface

I would like to welcome you to the Dx/Rx: Oncology series, a handbook series dedicated to the practical management of patients with common malignancies. This is the second edition of the Lung Cancer volume, and contains many important updates that are critical to the current management of lung cancer. In the first portion of the handbook, Dr. Azzoli provides important epidemiologic information about the role of cigarette smoking in lung cancer carcinogenesis, and provides an update of the National Lung Screening Trial that details the context within which lung cancer screening is effective. Dr. Azzoli expertly gives us an insight into the future of oncology—personalized medicine—within the context of the molecular biology of lung cancer. This includes highlights of not only EGFR mutations, but also novel discoveries of ALK mutations and their implications for therapy. The updated Rx section provides a nice algorithm for lung cancer treatment, including integration of molecularly-targeted approaches. Finally, Dr. Azzoli concludes with an update for 2012 that highlights the recent progress in the diagnosis and management of this deadly disease. It is therefore without hesitation that I am able to highly recommend this handbook—I trust you will find Dr. Azzoli's synopsis thoughtful and concise, and imminently user friendly. This handbook remains an important part of the Dx/Rx: Oncology series, and an exemplary representation of the success of the series.

Manish A. Shah, MD

Acknowledgments

I am grateful to Maureen Zakowski, MD, for providing photomicrographs for this text, and to my mentor, Mark Kris, MD, for teaching me all that I know about lung cancer.

Introduction

Lung cancer is the deadliest form of cancer, killing more people every year than breast, colon, and prostate cancers combined. It is also the most preventable cancer, with more than 85% of cases attributable to cigarette smoking. It is hard to imagine an advance in the diagnosis or treatment of lung cancer that could save as many lives as stopping people from smoking cigarettes or preventing them from smoking in the first place.

The cause-and-effect relationship between smoking and lung cancer has led to a stigmatization of patients with lung cancer. This is especially tragic because more than 20,000 Americans per year develop lung cancer having never smoked, and more than 70,000 former smokers still develop the disease each year, despite their efforts to quit. In fact, the majority of patients who develop lung cancer in the United States are ex-smokers.

A new frontier in the treatment of lung cancer is screening patients who are at risk for the disease in order to detect lung cancer at an early stage. In 2010, the results of a randomized study released by the United States National Cancer Institute showed that CT scans used to detect lung cancer early, before the onset of symptoms, can decrease risk of death from lung cancer in current or former cigarette smokers who are at the highest risk of developing lung cancer. A sobering outcome of this study is that, even in the population of smokers screened early for lung cancer, more than half who are diagnosed with lung cancer still die of this disease.

Clearly, far more can be accomplished in terms of public health and safety by decreasing the prevalence of cigarette smoking in America and around the world. Currently, more than 40 million Americans are active smokers, and if they care about their health, they should all quit smoking. The task of our generation of healthcare workers is to teach the dangers of cigarette smoking to all of our patients, to prevent them and their families from ever smoking, and to get current smokers to quit. It is never too late to quit. In fact, patients with lung cancer who manage to quit smoking live longer and tolerate their treatment better than patients who continue to smoke. But even if cigarettes were to disappear from the face of the Earth today, lung cancer would remain the most important cancer problem in our lifetimes because of the damage already done.

Lung cancer has a terrible reputation, in that the majority of patients who develop lung cancer eventually die of their disease. Hope lies in the fact that, even if it is not curable, lung cancer is treatable at any stage, and these treatments have been shown to improve both quality and length of life in patients with lung cancer. This text reviews important aspects of the diagnosis and treatment of patients with lung cancer. There are also two sections on other important cancers of the chest—mesothelioma and thymoma—which must be considered in the differential diagnosis of lung cancer.

Christopher G. Azzoli, MD

Notice

We have made every attempt to summarize accurately and concisely a multitude of references. However, the reader is reminded that times and medical knowledge change, transcription or understanding error is always possible, and crucial details can be omitted whenever such a comprehensive distillation as this is attempted in limited space. The primary purpose of this compilation is to cite literature on various sides of controversial issues; knowing where "truth" lies is usually difficult. We cannot, therefore, guarantee that every bit of information is absolutely accurate or complete. The reader should affirm that cited recommendations are still reasonable by reading the original articles and checking other sources, including local consultants as well as recent literature, before applying them.

Drugs and medical devices are discussed that may have limited availability controlled by the Food and Drug Administration (FDA) for use only in a research study or clinical trial. The drug information presented has been derived from reference sources, recently published data, and pharmaceutical tests. Research, clinical practice, and government regulations often change the accepted standard in this field. When consideration is being given to use of any drug in the clinical setting, the clinician or reader is responsible for determining FDA status of the drug; reading the package insert; and prescribing information for the most up-to-date recommendations on dose, precautions, and contraindications when determining the appropriate usage for the product. This is especially important in the case of drugs that are new or seldom used.

CHAPTER 1

Epidemiology

■ Smoking Tobacco Cigarettes Is Deadly

■ Lung cancer kills more Americans every year than any other type of cancer. The American Cancer Society (ACS) estimates there were 222,520 new cases of lung cancer in the United States in 2010, with 157,300 deaths attributable to lung cancer. This equals more deaths from lung cancer than colorectal, breast, and prostate cancers combined.[1]

■ Between 80% and 90% of all lung cancer can be attributed to cigarette smoking. The rising incidence of lung cancer from 1930 to the late 1980s mirrors the rise in popularity of cigarette smoking over the same time period.

■ Cigar and pipe smoking also increase the possibility of developing lung cancer; however, the risk of these is lower due to differences in smoking frequency and depth of inhalation.[2]

■ Cigarette Smoking in the United States

■ In 2009, the US Centers for Disease Control and Prevention (CDC) sponsored the National Health and Nutrition Examination Survey (NHANES), in which Americans were polled to estimate smoking prevalence in the United States. The results showed an estimated 40 million American adults actively smoking, and another 37 million former smokers.[3]

■ The risk of developing lung cancer is proportional to the number of packs of cigarettes smoked per day and the number of years of active smoking.

■ An efficient way to quantify a person's risk of developing lung cancer is to multiply the number of packs of cigarettes smoked per day by the number of years of active smoking. This statistic is known as "pack-years."

■ Most Americans are light smokers, with a cumulative habit of less than one pack of cigarettes per day for 15 years

(15 pack-years). About 15% are heavy smokers with a habit of over 30 pack-years.

■ Half of all ever smokers are former smokers. Despite quitting, these individuals remain at increased risk for developing lung cancer throughout their lifetime.

■ There is controversy as to what level of smoking constitutes a high enough risk of developing lung cancer to merit screening an asymptomatic person for the presence of lung cancer.

• The definition of "high risk" is a matter of debate.

• The National Lung Screening Trial, which randomized 50,000 American smokers to screening with computed tomography (CT) scan versus chest radiograph (CXR), defined a high risk of lung cancer as patients between the ages of 55 and 74 with at least a 30 pack-year history of cigarette smoking.[4]

■ Some estimates indicate that up to 20% of ever smokers develop lung cancer at some time in their lives.

■ Health-conscious tobacco policies and increased awareness of the dangers of smoking among Americans are lowering the rate of smoking in the United States. However, the rising popularity of cigarette smoking in the Third World portends a global epidemic of lung cancer in the next century unless global tobacco policies are changed.

■ Lung Cancer in US Women

■ Cigarette smoking gained popularity among women in the latter half of the 20th century. As a result of these smoking trends, the incidence of lung cancer in US women has increased sixfold over the last 40 years and is considered a contemporary epidemic.[5]

■ In 1987, lung cancer surpassed breast cancer as the leading cause of cancer death in US women.[1]

■ Although smoking prevalence among men has decreased by nearly 50% since the 1960s, smoking prevalence in women has decreased by only 25% during the same period. The social concept that cigarette smoking portrays maturity and independence, or may help to control weight, may make smoking especially appealing to young women.[6]

- There is controversy as to whether cigarette smoking is more dangerous for women than for men, with epidemiologic data available to support both sides of the argument.
  - This may be due to the fact that measuring cigarette smoke intake is dependent on whether the subject is a man or a woman (e.g., women may report their smoking habits more reliably than men).
  - Nevertheless, there are important biologic differences between men and women in their metabolism of tobacco carcinogens and in their hormone milieu, which may translate into a higher susceptibility to the cancer-causing effects of tobacco smoke among women.
- Female sex is associated with longer survival in patients with lung cancer, a fact that may reflect basic biologic differences between lung cancers in men and women.[5,7]
- Some authors have suggested that, with the rising number of cases of lung cancer in women, there is a "sex migration" in contemporary clinical trials, so that overall survival is improving over time due to the higher proportion of women enrolled.[8] Sex migration, like stage migration, should be taken into account when making historical comparisons between clinical trials.

■ Other Risk Factors for the Development of Lung Cancer

- Exposure to environmental tobacco smoke (ETS), also called "passive smoke," or "second-hand smoke," is another risk factor for developing lung cancer.[9]
  - This relationship was first observed in the nonsmoking spouses of heavy smokers.[10,11]
  - ETS may account for more than 3000 deaths per year in the United States.[12]
  - The fact that ETS results in a much lower exposure to tobacco smoke carcinogens than does active smoking yet is still strongly associated with lung cancer suggests that there is no threshold at which exposure to tobacco smoke may cause lung cancer.[2] This reinforces the importance of never smoking.

- The association of ETS with the development of lung cancer in adults, as well as the development of asthma and pneumonia in children, has influenced public policy and the banning of tobacco smoke in public areas to protect nonsmokers and children from ETS.

■ Radon (elemental symbol, Rn, atomic weight, 86) is a colorless, odorless, radioactive gas released from compounds in the soil. Exposure to radon is a risk factor for developing lung cancer.

- Although radon exposure increases a person's risk of developing lung cancer, the threshold of radon exposure and lung cancer risk is not known. In other words, it is unclear how much is too much.

- Radon levels in homes are measured in "picocuries per liter of air," or "pCi/L." In the United States, the average indoor radon level is 1.3 pCi/L. The average outdoor level is about 0.4 pCi/L.

- People who smoke cigarettes have a higher risk of developing radon-associated lung cancer.

- Home radon test kits are available in hardware stores and other retail outlets. Professional testing services are also available.

- Whether the level of radon in a home is too high, and what can or should be done to prevent radon from entering a home, is a matter of debate. More information is available from the US Environmental Protection Agency (http://www.epa.gov/radon/).

■ Coincident exposure to asbestos and tobacco smoke is a risk factor for developing lung cancer.

- Asbestos exposure is more directly associated with the development of another type of cancer, malignant pleural mesothelioma.

- Most people with a history of asbestos exposure who have gone on to develop lung cancer also smoked cigarettes. Therefore, a direct causal link between asbestos and lung cancer is lacking. However, individuals who smoke cigarettes and are also exposed to asbestos have a greater than additive increased risk of developing lung cancer.

- Asbestos is the name given to naturally occurring silicate minerals mined from rock and soil to be used as inflammable building material. Asbestos has been used for centuries as a fire-proofing material or insulation. The use of asbestos skyrocketed during the industrial revolution of the 19th and early 20th centuries.

* Inhaled asbestos crystals irritate the lungs and may cause a lung disease called asbestosis, in which diffuse, fibrous changes in the lungs result in progressive shortness of breath that may progress even after exposure to asbestos has stopped.

* Despite efforts to remove asbestos from building materials over the last 30 years, there are still an estimated 8 million Americans living with a history of significant asbestos exposure. Based on recent trends, the incidence of mesothelioma may have peaked in the U.S. in the last decade.

■ Does Lung Cancer Run in Families?

▧ Smoking habits tend to be shared within families, and second-hand smoke is also a risk factor, which may account for some observed familial associations.

▧ There is a genetic basis to how tobacco smoke is metabolized by an individual.[13] These genetic "polymorphisms" for the detoxification and metabolism of tobacco smoke may account for certain smokers developing lung cancer or emphysema while others appear to smoke with impunity.

▧ Recent studies of gene polymorphisms in lung cancer patients suggests that a specific genetic change in the nicotine receptor may increase susceptibility to lung cancer.[14] It is unknown whether this genetic predisposition increases the chance of developing lung cancer directly or indirectly by increasing the chance of nicotine dependence, thereby increasing exposure to tobacco smoke.

▧ One bona fide heritable lung cancer syndrome is a germline mutation in exon 20 of the epidermal growth factor receptor (EGFR), which is a change from threonine to methionine at position 790 (so-called EGFR T790M). Several families have been identified and reported with germline EGFR T790M and strong family histories of lung cancer.[15] This familial cancer syndrome is extremely rare, thus very little is known about the lifelong risk of developing lung cancer in people who carry this gene and whether they should be screened for lung cancer. Given the genetic basis for tobacco smoke metabolism and some emerging evidence of genetic predisposition to lung cancer that may run in families, any person with a first-degree relative (i.e., parent, sibling, child) with a smoking-related malignancy may be at higher risk for developing a smoking-related malignancy and should, therefore, be encouraged to abstain from cigarette smoking.

■ Lung Cancer in Never Smokers

■ Never smokers are more likely to develop a type of lung cancer called adenocarcinoma.

■ Persons who never smoked and have no history of exposure to second-hand tobacco smoke have no risk of developing small cell lung cancer (SCLC). If a never smoker is ever diagnosed with SCLC, serious consideration should be paid to the possibility that the diagnosis is incorrect.

■ Accumulated evidence demonstrates that patients with lung cancer who never smoked live longer than patients with smoking-related lung cancer.[16,17] In addition, never smokers are more likely to have druggable genetic mutations such as EGFR mutation and anaplastic lymphoma kinase (ALK) translocation than former or current smokers with lung cancer. In other words, lung cancer in never smokers may be genetically distinct from smoking-related lung cancer and is more likely to be treatable with targeted chemotherapy drugs.

■ Lung Cancer in Active Smokers

■ Once a patient has been diagnosed with lung cancer, smoking cessation remains important to his or her health and wellbeing and should be encouraged.

■ Studies suggest that patients who manage to quit smoking following their diagnosis of lung cancer live longer and tolerate their treatments better than patients who continue to smoke.[18,19]

■ CT Screening for Lung Cancer

■ Lung cancer is more likely to be cured if diagnosed at an early stage.

■ Recently, the results of the National Lung Screening Trial have shown that screening for lung cancer using CT scan reduces mortality due to lung cancer compared to screening with CXR.[20]

■ More than 50 years of randomized trials, involving more than 60,000 patients, failed to demonstrate the utility of screening with CXR or sputum cytology in reducing lung cancer mortality.

■ CT is more sensitive than CXR in detecting small lung tumors. This increased sensitivity results in a higher rate of discovery of both malignant and benign lung nodules compared to CXR.

■ CT scans involve a higher dose of radiation than CXR, and there is concern regarding cost effectiveness and risk of biopsy or surgery for the management of the many benign lung nodules discovered by CT.

■ Low-dose, helical chest CT scanning has long been of interest as a screening tool.

  • One nonrandomized trial used low-dose, helical chest CT scans to screen 1000 people 60 years of age or older with a 10 or greater pack-year history of smoking and detected 27 lung cancers, 85% of which were stage I.[21]

  • In addition to the cancers, 233 noncalcified nodules were detected that required close follow-up or biopsy.[21]

■ Between 2002 and 2004, the National Lung Screening Trial (NLST) enrolled 53,454 American smokers who did not have symptoms of lung cancer, and randomized them to three annual screening chest CT scans versus three annual CXRs.[20,22] Only individuals at the highest risk of developing lung cancer were eligible. High risk was defined as:

  • Age 55–74 years

  • Current or former smoker with at least a 30 pack-year history (one pack of cigarettes per day for 30 years, or two packs per day for 15 years, etc.)

- In the NLST, CT scans detected twice as many lung cancers as CXR (649/25,000 screened by CT versus 279/25,000 screened with CXR).

- CT scans also detected more abnormalities; 24% of individuals screened with CT had an abnormal finding, defined as a solid nodule greater than 4 millimeters in size or enlarged lymph nodes. Only 7% of CXRs were abnormal. A total of 96.4% of the positive screening results in the low-dose CT group were false-positive results.

- Participants were followed from 2004 to 2010. Final results showed that individuals screened with CT scan were 20% less likely to die of lung cancer compared to individuals screened with CXR (356 lung cancer deaths in the CT arm, 443 lung cancer deaths in the CXR arm).[20]

- In addition, all-cause mortality was reduced in the CT arm by 7% (1877 total deaths in the CT arm, 2000 total deaths in the CXR arm). The reason for the reduction in all-cause mortality is uncertain, but reassuring that extra tests, biopsies, and surgeries that occurred in the CT arm to manage all of the benign lung nodules discovered by CT did not result in increased mortality.

- The final decision as to whether or not a patient should be screened for lung cancer remains in the hands of the individual healthcare practitioner.

- Based on current data, it is reasonable to pursue CT screening of asymptomatic persons who meet the enrollment criteria of the NLST.[20]

- In addition, any person with a history of a prior smoking-related malignancy has an even higher risk of developing a new primary lung cancer than the patients enrolled in the NLST. As such, it is also reasonable to screen patients with a history of lung cancer to detect new lung cancers at an earlier stage.

- Any asymptomatic patient who is screened for lung cancer should be made aware that false-positive results may prompt biopsies or the need for additional follow-up scans, leading to potentially unnecessary risk, cost, and worry.

■ References

1. Jemal A, Bray F, Center MM, et al. Global cancer statistics. *CA Cancer J Clin.* 2011;61(2):69–90.

2. Alberg AJ, Ford, JG, Samet JM; American College of Chest Physicians. Epidemiology of lung cancer: ACCP evidence-based clinical practice guidelines (2nd edition). *Chest.* 2007; 32(3):29S-55S.

3. Centers for Disease Control and Prevention. *Vital Signs: Current Cigarette Smoking Among Adults Aged ≥ 18 Years—United States, 2009.* Morbidity and Mortality Weekly Report 2010;59(35):1135–1140

4. National Lung Screening Trial Research Team, Aberle DR, Adams AM, Berg CD, et al. Reduced lung-cancer mortality with low-dose computed tomographic screening. *N Engl J Med.* 2011 Aug 4;365(5):395–409.

5. de Perrot M, Licker M, Bouchardy C, et al. Sex differences in presentation, management, and prognosis of patients with non-small cell lung carcinoma. *J Thorac Cardiovasc Surg.* 2000;119(1):21–26.

6. Patel JD, Bach PB, Kris MG. Lung cancer in US women: a contemporary epidemic. *JAMA.* 2004;291(14):1763–1768.

7. Ouellette D, Desbiens G, Emond C, et al. Lung cancer in women compared with men: stage, treatment, and survival. *Ann Thorac Surg.* 1998;66(4):1140–1143; discussion 1143–1144.

8. Patel JD, Kris MG, Venkatraman E, et al. Collateral damage from the lung cancer explosion in American women: has sex migration replaced stage migration as a confounding factor in lung cancer trials? *Lung Cancer* [abstract O-207]. 2003; 41(suppl 2):S61.

9. Respiratory health effects of passive smoking: lung cancer and other disorders. Washington, D.C.: US Environmental Protection Agency (EPA); 1992. Report No.: 600/006F.

10. Hirayama T. Non-smoking wives of heavy smokers have a higher risk of lung cancer: a study from Japan. *Br Med J (Clin Res Ed).* 1981;282(6259):183–185.

11. Trichopoulos D, Kalandidi A, Sparros L, et al. Lung cancer and passive smoking. *Int J Cancer.* 1981;27(1):1–4.

12. Respiratory health effects of passive smoking: lung cancer and other disorders. Washington, D.C.: US Environmental Protection Agency (EPA); 1992. Report No.: 600/006F.

13. Hecht SS. Tobacco smoke carcinogens and lung cancer. *J Natl Cancer Inst.* 1999;91(14):1194–1210.

14. Hung RJ, McKay JD, Gaborieau V, et al. A susceptibility locus for lung cancer maps to nicotinic acetylcholine receptor subunit genes on 15q25. *Nature.* 2008;452(7187):633–637.

15. Girard N, Lou E, Azzoli CG, et al. Analysis of genetic variants in never-smokers with lung cancer facilitated by an

Internet-based blood collection protocol: a preliminary report. *Clin Cancer Res.* 2010;16(2):755–763.

16. Janjigian YY, McDonnell K, Kris MG, et al. Pack-years of cigarette smoking as a prognostic factor in patients with stage IIIB/IV nonsmall cell lung cancer. *Cancer.* 2010;116(3):670–675.

17. Kawaguchi T, Takada M, Kubo A, et al. Performance status and smoking status are independent favorable prognostic factors for survival in non-small cell lung cancer: a comprehensive analysis of 26,957 patients with NSCLC. *J Thorac Oncol.* 2010;5(5):620–630.

18. Videtic GM, Stitt LW, Dar AR, et al. Continued cigarette smoking by patients receiving concurrent chemoradiotherapy for limited-stage small-cell lung cancer is associated with decreased survival. *J Clin Oncol.* 2003;21(8):1544–1549.

19. Fox JL, Rosenzweig KE, Ostroff JS. The effect of smoking status on survival following radiation therapy for non-small cell lung cancer. *Lung Cancer.* 2004;44(3):287–293.

20. National Lung Screening Trial Research Team, Aberle DR, Adams AM, Berg CD, Black WC, et al. Reduced lung-cancer mortality with low-dose computed tomographic screening. *N Engl J Med.* 2011 Aug 4;365(5):395–409.

21. Henschke CI, Yankelevitz DF, Libby DM, et al. International Early Lung Cancer Action Program Investigators. Survival of patients with stage I lung cancer detected on CT screening. *N Engl J Med.* 2006;355(17):1763–1771.

22. Aberle DR, Berg CD, Black WC, et al.; National Lung Screening Trial Research Team. The National Lung Screening Trial: overview and study design. *Radiol.* 2011;258(1):243–253.

CHAPTER 2

Histopathology of Lung Cancer

■ Diagnosis Requires a Tissue Biopsy

■ The key to the diagnosis of lung cancer is the examination of biopsy tissue by a pathologist. Lung cancer is categorized by its appearance under the microscope.

■ Optimal histologic classification of lung cancer, and molecular testing, demands more material in a diagnostic biopsy than what is obtained in a routine cytology specimen.[1]

• Surgical biopsies or core needle biopsies are preferred to give the pathologist more material to study the morphology and architecture of the tumor for histologic classification.

• Additional material allows molecular studies to be performed on the tissue to check for gene mutations, or translocations, which may influence selection of chemotherapy.

• As such, if fine needle aspirate is the only option to obtain diagnostic tissue, a more generous aspirate or multiple aspirates should be performed to obtain sufficient material to make a cell block for future molecular testing.[2]

■ Small Cell Lung Cancer

■ Certain lung tumors are made up of small, round cells with large nuclei that turn blue when stained with hematoxylin and eosin (H&E). This type of lung cancer, called oat cell or small cell lung cancer (SCLC), is a distinct clinical entity from other types of lung cancer (see **Figure 2.1**).

■ SCLC tends to grow rapidly and is more likely to spread throughout the body (metastasize), making it less amenable

11

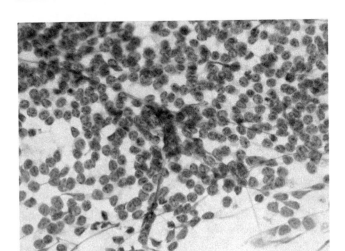

Figure 2.1 Small cell carcinoma (cytologic preparation).

to treatment with surgery. Almost all patients with SCLC require treatment with chemotherapy.

■ SCLC arises from neuroendocrine cells within the lung that express proteins on their surface consistent with this phenotype, including synaptophysin, chromogranin, and neuron-specific enolase.

■ SCLC is so strongly associated with cigarette smoking or exposure to second-hand tobacco smoke that a diagnosis of SCLC in a never smoker or someone without any exposure to environmental tobacco smoke should be called into question.

  • Other small, round, blue cell tumors include certain types of sarcoma, such as Ewing's sarcoma of the chest wall (Askin tumor), primitive neuroectodermal tumor (PNET), and rhabdomyosarcoma.

  • Melanoma and carcinoid tumors may also masquerade as SCLC.

■ Carcinoid Tumor of the Lung

■ There are tumors that arise in the lung with neuroendocrine phenotype that, unlike SCLC, grow slowly, rarely metastasize, and are treatable with surgery alone. These so-called "carcinoid" tumors of the lung are also made up of small, round, blue cells but can be distinguished from SCLC by their low-grade appearance and lack of mitotic figures.

- Carcinoid tumors tend to be highly resistant to chemotherapy and radiation therapy and are best treated with surgery.

- More aggressive carcinoid tumors with an intermediate number of mitotic figures are known as atypical carcinoids.

  - Compared with typical carcinoids, atypical carcinoids grow faster and have a higher potential for metastasis. They are also potentially more responsive to radiation or chemotherapy.

  - Although surgical resection of atypical carcinoids is preferred, these tumors behave in a fashion intermediate between SCLC and typical carcinoids, and may merit treatment with radiation or chemotherapy.

- Large cell tumors that express neuroendocrine tumor markers suggest an association with SCLC. However, large cell neuroendocrine tumors are less responsive to chemotherapy than SCLC and are treated as non-small cell tumors.

■ Non–Small Cell Lung Cancer

- All other types of lung cancer are, by convention, categorized as non-small cell lung cancer (NSCLC). NSCLC has a variety of histopathologic appearances, which are listed in **Table 2.1**. All varieties of NSCLC are potentially treatable with surgery.

- The majority of NSCLC tumors are carcinomas, believed to arise from lung epithelial cells. NSCLC tends to express cytokeratins in a distinct pattern (positive for CK7, negative for CK20).

- Clinically relevant subgroups of NSCLC are being discovered, and the designation NSCLC is slowly being replaced by more specific terminology.

Table 2.1 Histologic Subtypes of Lung Cancer

1. Carcinoid / atypical carcinoid of lung

2. Small cell carcinoma

3. Non-small cell carcinoma
   a. Adenocarcinoma
      Descriptive subtypes:
         i. Nonmucinous vs. mucinous
         ii. Papillary
         iii. Micropapillary
         iv. Acinar
         v. Invasive vs. in situ
         vi. Lepidic vs. solid
         vii. Adenosquamous (mixed)
   b. Squamous carcinoma
   c. Large cell carcinoma
   d. Large cell neuroendocrine carcinoma
   e. Sarcomatoid carcinoma
   f. Undifferentiated / unspecified carcinoma / other

4. Secondary neoplasms metastatic to lung

- Adenocarcinoma, the most common form of NSCLC, is the type of lung cancer least closely associated with cigarette smoking.
  - As cigarette smoking rates decline in the United States, there is an increasing preponderance of adenocarcinoma among all types of lung cancer. In Europe and Asia, adenocarcinoma is less predominant.
  - Adenocarcinomas most often arise in the periphery of the lung parenchyma from epithelial cells involved in gland formation.
  - Adenocarcinomas may grow in acinar, papillary, micopapillary, lepidic, or solid growth patterns and are often associated with the production of mucin (see **Figure 2.2**).
- Lepidic growth refers to growth of cancer cells along the lining of alveolar spaces and airways. A classical term for lepidic growth is bronchioloalveolar carcinoma (BAC). Recent changes in classification of lung adenocarcinoma

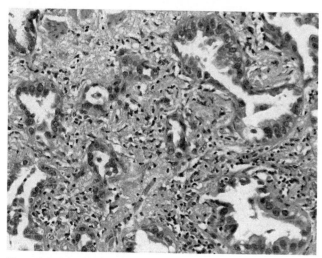

Figure 2.2 Adenocarcinoma.

have made the term BAC obsolete and potentially mislead-
ing (see **Figure 2.3**).[1]

- Some lung tumors have features of both invasive adenocarcinoma and BAC. Other tumors are pure BAC
  without invasion. Since the term BAC alone does not
  distinguish pure from mixed tumors, a new term for
  pure BAC, so-called adenocarcinoma in situ, has been
  adopted. All other tumors should be considered invasive adenocarcinomas regardless of BAC component.[1]
- Atypical adenomatous hyperplasia (AAH) is a benign,
  perhaps premalignant, lung lesion characterized by a
  proliferation of cells along alveolar septae that does not
  meet the criteria for adenocarcinoma in situ. AAH typically does not cause radiologic changes and is therefore
  most often found incidentally in a lung specimen resected for some other reason.
- Lung adenocarcinoma in situ is less likely to spread
  through the blood to distant sites in the body than other
  types of NSCLC; however, it may spread within the
  lungs from lobe to lobe, perhaps via the airways.
- Lung adenocarcinoma in situ and/or with lepidic growth
  often take on the appearance of "ground glass" on

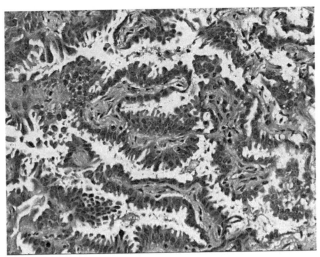

Figure 2.3 Adenocarcinoma with lepidic growth (formerly known as bronchioloalveolar carcinoma).

computed tomography (CT) scans because of the presence of air within the tumor. BAC tumors may also generate mucin, which can fill air spaces and result in consolidation of an entire lobe of the lung; this is known as the "pneumonic" form of lung adenocarcinoma.
- Perhaps due to the presence of air within the tumor, adenocarcinoma in situ is less likely to light up on FDG-PET scans than other types of adenocarcinoma.
- Adenocarcinoma in situ rarely spreads outside of the lung and is among the slowest growing types of lung cancer. As such, patients with multifocal, small ground-glass opacities may be followed without the need for surgery, or undergo multiple small surgeries to remove serial lung cancers with good long-term survival.
- Squamous cell carcinoma is a type of NSCLC with characteristics of squamous epithelium—namely, keratin formation, intercellular bridging, and solid (nonglandular) appearance. Squamous tumors tend to arise near the center of the chest, within major bronchi, and are more commonly associated with cigarette smoking than adenocarcinoma (see **Figure 2.4**).

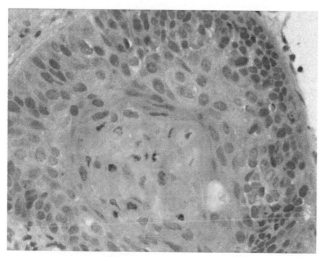

Figure 2.4 Squamous cell carcinoma.

* Patients with squamous carcinoma are less likely to benefit from treatment with the drug pemetrexed (Alimta), and more likely to develop hemoptysis after treatment with the drug bevacizumab (Avastin). These drugs are preferentially given to patients with stage IV NSCLC that is not squamous.
* As a result of these implications for drug selection, it is increasingly important to classify NSCLC as squamous, adenocarcinoma, or other.[1]
* In those cases where a specimen shows NSCLC lacking either definite squamous or adenocarcinoma morphology, or in a small biopsy or cytology specimen, immunohistochemistry may be used to refine the diagnosis.[1]
    * Thyroid transcription factor 1 (TTF-1) can help confirm the cancer is of lung origin.
    * p63 is a reliable marker for squamous histology and CK5/6 also can be useful.
    * Cytokeratin 7 tends to stain adenocarcinoma more often than squamous cell carcinoma.
    * Cases positive for TTF-1 and/or mucin with a negative squamous marker are often classified as "NSCLC favor adenocarcinoma."

- Cases that are positive for a squamous marker, with at least moderate, diffuse staining, and a negative adenocarcinoma marker and/or mucin stains, are often classified as "NSCLC favor squamous cell carcinoma."[1]
- Molecular profiling of NSCLC by RNA expression recapitulates histopathologic categorization.[3,4] Despite these advances in molecular diagnostics, histopathology remains the most important factor for the diagnosis and treatment of lung cancer. This may change in the future as more is discovered about genetic fingerprints that may predict sensitivity to specific types of chemotherapy.
- Adenosquamous carcinoma has features of both adenocarcinoma and squamous carcinoma, often with solid nests of cells as well as gland formation. These mixed histology tumors suggest that different NSCLC phenotypes may share similar genetic changes.
- Large cell carcinoma lacks features of adenocarcinoma and squamous carcinoma and is considered a more poorly differentiated form of NSCLC.
  - Large cell tumors that express mucin are more related to adenocarcinoma.
  - Large cell tumors that express neuroendocrine tumor markers suggest an association with SCLC. Large cell neuroendocrine tumors are far less responsive to chemotherapy than SCLC and carry a poor prognosis compared with other types of NSCLC.[5]
  - Retrospective case series of patients with large cell neuroendocrine tumors treated with surgery show higher rates of recurrence and death even after successful surgery. These series suggest the need for more aggressive use of post-operative chemotherapy (adjuvant chemotherapy) for this histologic subtype.[6–8]
- Some NSCLC tumors demonstrate features of sarcoma, namely, spindle-shaped or pleomorphic cells, which can make them easy to confuse with true sarcoma.
  - These so-called sarcomatoid carcinomas are treated the same as all NSCLC tumors, that is with surgical removal if possible.

* Chemotherapy drugs useful for the treatment of NSCLC, rather than sarcoma-specific drugs, are often used to treat sarcomatoid NSCLC.

Secondary Neoplasms Metastatic to the Lung

* Primary lung cancer should not be confused with other cancers that have spread to the lung from elsewhere in the body, or so-called secondary lung tumors. This is vitally important in prescribing treatment.
  * Breast or prostate cancers metastatic to the lung may be treatable with hormonal therapy.
  * Thyroid cancer metastatic to the lung may be treatable with surgery or radioactive iodine.
  * Germ cell tumors, gastrointestinal tumors, renal cell cancer, melanoma, or lymphoma growing in the lung may respond to different chemotherapies than NSCLC.
  * Adenoid cystic carcinoma, a salivary gland tumor that often spreads to the lung, is best left untreated due to its indolent growth pattern.
* In addition to histopathology, the physician making the diagnosis of lung cancer must take into account the patient's symptoms, physical examination, medical history, the appearance of the tumor on radiologic scans, and risk factors for lung cancer. If, after these considerations, the physician is still not sure where a carcinoma started, he or she may give a diagnosis of metastatic carcinoma of unknown primary (CUP).
* Most treatments for metastatic CUP are the same as those for metastatic NSCLC.

References

1. Travis WD, Brambilla E, Noguchi M, et al. International association for the study of lung cancer/American thoracic society/European respiratory society international multidisciplinary classification of lung adenocarcinoma. *J Thorac Oncol.* 2011; 6(2):244–285.
2. Azzoli CG, Baker S Jr, Termin S, et al. American Society of Clinical Oncology Clinical Practice Guideline update on

chemotherapy for stage IV non–small-cell lung cancer. *J Clin Oncol.* 2009;27(36):6251–6266.

3. Bhattacharjee A, Richards WG, Staunton J, et al. Classification of human lung carcinomas by mRNA expression profiling reveals distinct adenocarcinoma subclasses. *Proc Natl Acad Sci USA.* 2001;98(24):13790–13795.

4. Beer DG, Kardia SL, Huang CC, et al. Gene-expression profiles predict survival of patients with lung adenocarcinoma. *Nat Med.* 2002;8(8):816–824.

5. Rossi G, Cavazza A, Marchioni A, et al. Role of chemotherapy and the receptor tyrosine kinases KIT, PDGFRalpha, PDGFRbeta, and Met in large-cell neuroendocrine carcinoma of the lung. *J Clin Oncol.* 2005;23(34):8774–8785.

6. Saji, H, Tsuboi M, Matsubayashi J, et al. Clinical response of large cell neuroendocrine carcinoma of the lung to perioperative adjuvant chemotherapy. *Anticancer Drugs.* 2010;21(1):89–93.

7. Iyoda A, Hiroshima K, Moriya Y, et al. Postoperative recurrence and the role of adjuvant chemotherapy in patients with pulmonary large-cell neuroendocrine carcinoma. *J Thorac Cardiovasc Surg.* 2009;138(2):446–453.

8. Iyoda A, Hiroshima K, Toyozaki T, et al. Adjuvant chemotherapy for large cell carcinoma with neuroendocrine features. *Cancer.* 2001;92(5):1108–1112.

CHAPTER 3

Molecular Biology of Lung Cancer

■ Cigarette Smoking and Genetic Mutations

■ More than 20 carcinogens have been identified in tobacco smoke. The most prominent carcinogens are 4-(methylnitrosamino)-1-(3-pyridyl)-1-butanone and polycyclic aromatic hydrocarbons such as benzapyrene.[1] Free radicals and reactive oxygen species found in tobacco smoke also damage DNA.

• Carcinogens bind covalently to DNA, leading to miscoding of DNA and genetic mutations.

• Free radicals and reactive oxygen species result in DNA strand breaks, with resultant genetic mutations during DNA repair.

■ Nicotine is not carcinogenic but leads to smoking addiction, thereby increasing carcinogen exposure.

■ The carcinogens found in mainstream tobacco smoke are also found in second-hand smoke, albeit at lower concentrations.

■ Genetic differences exist among individuals in terms of metabolic activation of carcinogens as well as detoxification.

• Epidemiologic data suggest that genetic predispositions to lung cancer exist for all smoking-related malignancies.

• Recent studies of gene polymorphisms in lung cancer patients suggest that a specific genetic change in the nicotine receptor may increase susceptibility to lung cancer.[2] It is unknown whether this genetic predisposition increases the chance of developing lung cancer directly or indirectly by increasing the chance of nicotine dependence, thereby increasing exposure to tobacco smoke.

21

■ Anyone who has a first-degree relative with a smoking-related cancer should not smoke cigarettes.

■ Lung cancer is caused by a series of genetic changes in normal cells that result in abnormal growth and, ultimately, cell invasion and metastasis. These genetic changes include overactivity of oncogenes (genes that signal cells to grow and divide) as well as underactivity of tumor suppressor genes (genes that signal cells to stop growing or undergo apoptosis [programmed cell death]).

■ The genetic changes that cause lung cancer are acquired, either due to exposure to tobacco smoke or by chance.

   • One bona fide heritable lung cancer syndrome is a germline mutation in exon 20 of the epidermal growth factor receptor (EGFR), which is a change from threonine to methionine at position 790 (so-called EGFR T790M).

   • Several families have been identified and reported with germline EGFR T790M and strong family histories of lung cancer.[3] This familial cancer syndrome is extremely rare, and as such very little is known about the lifelong risk of developing lung cancer in people who carry this gene and whether they should be screened for lung cancer.

■ Oncogenes Implicated in Lung Cancer Carcinogenesis

■ EGFR/HER-1

   • Most NSCLC tumors express EGFR and its natural ligands, transforming growth factor alpha (TGF-a), amphiregulin, and epiregulin. EGFR regulates the growth of many different types of cells, both epithelial and nonepithelial.

      ■ EGFR was first identified as a proto-oncogene more than 20 years ago during studies of viruses that cause leukemia in chickens. The viral protein (v-erb-B) produces a constitutive EGFR signal in avian erythroblasts, resulting in their abnormal proliferation. Similarly, in human cells, the proto-oncogene EGFR can become an oncogene if a mutation in the coding sequence, or aberrant expression of the protein, results in amplification of the normal growth signal.

▪ EGFR is one of four related transmembrane glycoprotein receptors (human epidermal growth factor receptors)—HER-1 (which is EGFR), HER-2, HER-3, and HER-4.

▪ EGFR/HER-1 is a 170 kD protein that consists of an extracellular ligand-binding domain, a transmembrane region, a cytoplasmic protein tyrosine kinase domain, and a carboxy-terminal tail. Upon ligand binding (typically by TGF-a, or EGF), EGFR is able to undergo either homo- or heterodimerization with another family member followed by phosphorylation of tyrosine residues in the carboxy terminus of the receptor. These phosphorylated tyrosine residues serve as docking sites for a number of signal transduction and adaptor molecules, most of which are protein kinases.

▪ Some important signal transduction molecules downstream of EGFR signal include the PI3K→AKT pathway and the Ras→Raf→MEK pathway (see **Figure 3.1**).

▪ Drugs that inhibit the intracellular growth signal from EGFR/HER-1 are effective treatments for patients with NSCLC. The discovery of these drugs—including gefitinib (Iressa), erlotinib (Tarceva), and afatinib (Tomtovok) has resulted in increased interest in the EGFR signaling pathway as an important mechanism of NSCLC carcinogenesis.

▪ The mechanism by which the EGFR signal is upregulated in lung cancer is an area of active research.

• EGFR overexpression can be detected by immunohistochemistry in about one-third or more of all NSCLC tumors.[4,5]

• It appears that EGFR overexpression is more common in higher stage tumors and in squamous cell carcinomas as compared with adenocarcinomas and large cell carcinomas.

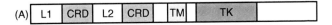

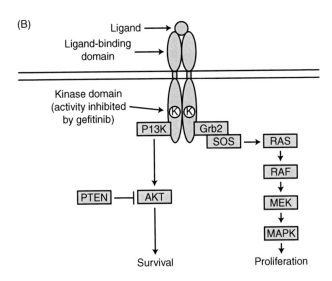

Figure 3.1 A: Schematic protein structure of EGFR. L1 and L2, ligand-binding domains; CRD, cysteine-rich domains; TM, transmembrane domain; TK, tyrosine kinase domain. **B:** Schematic of EGFR signaling pathways. **C:** Chemical structure of gefitinib, a competitive, reversible inhibitor of ATP at the TK domain of EGFR.

Adapted with permission from *Semin Cancer Biol*, Vol. 14, Pao W et al, Targeting the epidermal growth factor receptor tyrosine kinase with gefitinib (iressa) in non-small cell lung cancer (NSCLC), 33–40, Copyright Elsevier 2004.

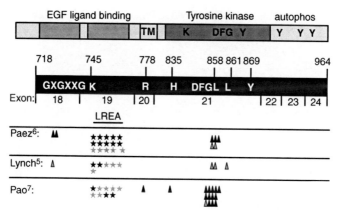

Figure 3.2 Summary of mutations discovered in non-small cell cancers as reported in 2004. The tyrosine kinase domain of EGFR is encoded by exons 18–24 (amino acids 718–964). The sites of described mutations are G719, L747–A750, S752, R776, H835, L858, and L861. Functional landmarks include the GXGXXG motif at position 719, the K745 critical for ATP binding, the DFG motif at position 855, and a tyrosine at 869.
Adapted with permission from Pao W, et al. EGF receptor gene mutations are common in lung cancers from "never smokers" and are associated with sensitivity of tumors to gefitinib and erlotinib. *Proc Natl Acad Sci USA.* 2004;101:13306–13311. Copyright 2004 National Academy of Sciences, USA.

- Gene amplification of EGFR has been identified in some NSCLC samples.
- A mutant receptor (EGFRvIII) has been identified in several cancers, including NSCLC. EGFRvIII is constitutively active, even in the absence of ligand.
- Activating mutations in the EGFR gene have been discovered in the NSCLC of patients who have responded to gefitinib and erlotinib.[6–8] These mutations are located in the catalytic kinase domain (ATP binding domain) of the EGFR protein. A summary of clinically important mutations is presented in **Figure 3.2**, and an illustrative clinical vignette in **Figure 3.3**.
- Patients with metastatic NSCLC and EGFR mutation have a much better prognosis than patients who

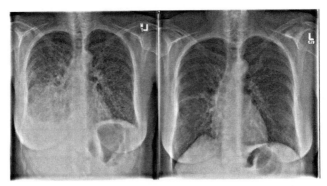

Figure 3.3 Patients whose cancer has an activating mutation in the catalytic kinase domain of EGFR may have dramatic responses to treatment with gefitinib or erlotinib. This patient had a documented EGFR exon 21 L858R mutation and had a dramatic radiologic and clinical response to gefitinib (250 mg oral daily tablet) that lasted for 10 months before the cancer started to grow again.

do not have EGFR mutation (median survival of 20–30 months instead of 10–12 months).[9]

- In addition, five prospective randomized trials in patients with metastatic, EGFR-mutant NSCLC have shown that gefitinib or erlotinib provide these patients with higher rates of radiologic response and longer progression-free interval compared to cytotoxic chemotherapy.[10–15]

- Gefitinib and erlotinib have fewer side effects than traditional chemotherapy.

- As a result of the importance of EGFR mutation in disease prognosis and for selection of optimal chemotherapy, testing for EGFR mutation is now considered a routine part of pathologic analysis of NSCLC tissue.

- NSCLC that at first responds to gefitinib or erlotinib eventually acquires resistance to these drugs and begins to grow again despite continued treatment. Genetic analysis of NSCLC with acquired resistance to these drugs has identified a second mutation in exon 20, which leads to substitution of methionine for threonine at position 790 (T790M) in the kinase domain and blocks the binding of drug to EGFR.[16,17]

* Patients with acquired resistance to erlotinib or gefitinib and EGFR T790M have a better prognosis than patients whose genetic mechanism for acquired resistance is unknown.[18]

* Acquired resistance may also be treatable, or preventable, once better understanding of the underlying molecular mechanism is achieved and better drugs become available. Given the prognostic importance of this discovery, patients with EGFR mutation and acquired resistance to gefitinib or erlotinib may undergo repeat biopsies to document EGFR T790M. The molecular mechanism of resistance may also inform clinical trial enrollment in new drugs designed to target these cancers.[19]

* K-ras

  * K-ras is a member of the ras gene family. Ras proteins are coupled to growth receptors on the surface of cells via protein-protein interactions.

    * Ras protein functions in normal cells to transduce growth signals from the cell membrane into the nucleus of the cell. The ras signal is active when ras is bound to guanosine triphosphate (GTP).

    * Normal ras hydrolyzes GTP to guanosine diphosphate (GDP), turning off the signal. Mutant K-ras results in constitutive growth signals from the cell membrane, even in the absence of signal from membrane receptors, with activation of the Ras→Raf→MEK signal transduction pathway.

    * Patients with stage IV NSCLC and K-ras mutation are unlikely to respond to treatment with EGFR tyrosine kinase inhibitors.

      * This is believed to be because the K-ras growth signal is downstream of EGFR so that blocking EGFR signal is not as helpful in these patients.

      * It is unknown whether K-ras mutation status predicts benefit from antibodies against EGFR (cetuximab [Erbitux]). This is for lack of data.

Cetuximab is not effective for the treatment of patients with advanced colorectal cancer and K-ras mutation.[20]

- ALK
  - Anaplastic lymphoma kinase (ALK) is a proto-oncogene growth kinase in the cytoplasm of cancer cells that becomes overactive due to translocations resulting in fusion genes. ALK fuses to the echinoderm microtubule-associated protein-like 4 (EML4), causing an excess of growth signal, enhanced cellular proliferation, survival, and changes in cell shape through KRAS-ERK, JAK3-STAT, and PI3-K pathways.[21]
    - Compared with non-ALK patients, patients with EML4-ALK mutant tumors tend to be younger, are more likely to be men, are more likely to be never or former light smokers, and tend to be adenocarcinomas (predominantly signet ring subtype).[22]
    - Patients with EML4-ALK translocation are resistant to EGFR tyrosine kinase inhibitors.[22]
    - A novel tyrosine kinase inhibitor specific to ALK (crizotinib, [Xalkori]) has shown promising activity in patients with metastatic NSCLC and ALK translocation in a phase 1 clinical trial. In 2011, the results of phase 2 clinical trials led to United States FDA approval of this drug for patients with ALK translocation.[23]
    - Like EGFR mutation testing, routine testing of NSCLC for ALK translocation in order to select optimal chemotherapy is now a standard of care.
    - ALK can be detected in NSCLC tumor tissue using fluorescent in situ hybridization (FISH), with PCR and immunohistochemical tests also in development.
- Myc
  - Members of the myc gene family are nuclear proteins that bind to DNA and stimulate expression of many genes required for cell cycle progression.
    - Myc overexpression, or gene amplification, is commonly found in lung cancers.

- The precise mechanism by which Myc overexpression contributes to lung tumor carcinogenesis is poorly understood, but it is believed to involve downstream effects on numerous cyclin-dependent kinases, which drive the cell cycle.

■ Tumor Suppressor Genes Implicated in Lung Cancer Carcinogenesis

- Rb
  - Rb protein controls whether a cell proceeds from normal growth to cell division (transition from G1→S phase of the cell cycle).
    - In normal cells, Rb is inactivated by phosphorylation and activated by dephosphorylation.
    - Active (dephosphorylated) Rb binds and inactivates the cellular transcription factor E2F1, which blocks cell cycle progression.
    - When Rb is inactivated by phosphorylation, E2F1 remains active and allows the cell to proceed from G1 into S phase.
    - Abnormalities or loss of Rb are a common genetic defect in lung cancers, especially SCLC.
- p16^{INK4a}
  - Also known as CDKN2A, this is another gene involved in control of the cell cycle, upstream of Rb.
    - p16^{INK4a} protein inhibits the protein kinases (CDK-4/6) that activate cyclin D1 and inactivate Rb by phosphorylation.
    - Loss of p16^{INK4a} function leads to loss of Rb function and inappropriate cell cycling.
- p53
  - The p53 gene is the most commonly mutated gene in human cancer.
    - About 60% of human lung cancers contain inactivating mutations in p53.
    - Normal p53 has several functions in the cell. It binds to DNA and can activate transcription of genes, which results in cell cycle arrest and apoptosis.

- When DNA damage occurs due to carcinogens such as those present in tobacco smoke, normal cells arrest at the G1-S cell cycle checkpoint until the damage is repaired.
- Cells that lack p53 or contain a mutant form do not arrest at G1.

■ Benzapyrene from tobacco smoke undergoes metabolic activation in the liver to a potent mutagen that causes G-to-T transversion mutations, resulting in inactivating mutations at codons 175, 248, and 273 of the p53 gene.

■ Once p53 is inactivated, cells may become even more susceptible to the DNA-damaging effects of tobacco smoke carcinogens.

■ FHIT
- Deletions on chromosome 3p are one of the most common genetic alterations found in lung cancers. The fragile histidine triad (FHIT) gene is located on the short arm of chromosome 3 (3p14.2), and FHIT protein is reduced or absent in the majority of lung cancers.
  ■ FHIT inactivation is twice as frequent in the tumors of smokers as in those of nonsmokers.[24]
  ■ The exact molecular mechanism of the FHIT protein remains unknown, but this is an area of active research.

■ References

1. Hecht SS. Tobacco smoke carcinogens and lung cancer. *J Natl Cancer Inst.* 1999;91(14):1194–1210.
2. Hung RJ, McKay JD, Gaborieau V, et al. A susceptibility locus for lung cancer maps to nicotinic acetylcholine receptor subunit genes on 15q25. *Nature.* 2008;452(7187): 633–637.
3. Girard N, LouE, Azzoli CG, et al. Analysis of genetic variants in never-smokers with lung cancer facilitated by an Internet-based blood collection protocol: a preliminary report. *Clin Cancer Res.* 2010;16(2):755–763.
4. Rusch V, Klimstra D, Venkatraman E, et al. Overexpression of the epidermal growth factor receptor and its ligand transforming growth factor alpha is frequent in resectable non-small cell lung cancer but does not predict tumor progression. *Clin Cancer Res.* 1997;3(4):515–522.

5. Pfeiffer P, Nexo E, Bentzen SM, et al. Enzyme-linked immuno-sorbent assay of epidermal growth factor receptor in lung cancer: comparisons with immunohistochemistry, clinicopathological features and prognosis. *Br J Cancer.* 1998;78(1):96–99.
6. Lynch TJ, Bell DW, Sordella R, et al. Activating mutations in the epidermal growth factor receptor underlying responsiveness of non-small-cell lung cancer to gefitinib. *N Engl J Med.* 2004;350(21):2129–2139.
7. Paez JG, Janne PA, Lee JC, et al. EGFR mutations in lung cancer: correlation with clinical response to gefitinib therapy." *Science.* 2004;304(5676):1497–1500.
8. Pao W, Miller V, Zakowski M, et al. EGF receptor gene mutations are common in lung cancers from "never smokers" and are associated with sensitivity of tumors to gefitinib and erlotinib. *Proc Natl Acad Sci US.* 2004;101(36):13306–13311.
9. Fukuoka M, Wu YL, Thongprasert S, et al. Biomarker analyses and final overall survival results from a phase III, randomized, open-label, first-line study of gefitinib versus carboplatin/paclitaxel in clinically selected patients with advanced non-small-cell lung cancer in Asia (IPASS). *J Clin Oncol.* 2011; 29(21):2866–2874.
10. Maemondo M, Inoue A, Kobayashi K, et al. Gefitinib or chemotherapy for non-small-cell lung cancer with mutated EGFR. *N Engl J Med.* 2010;362(25):2380–2388.
11. Mok TS, Wu YL, Thongprasert S, et al. Gefitinib or carboplatin-paclitaxel in pulmonary adenocarcinoma. *N Engl J Med.* 2009; 361(10):947–957.
12. Mitsudomi T, Morita S, Yatabe Y, et al. Gefitinib versus cisplatin plus docetaxel in patients with non-small-cell lung cancer harbouring mutations of the epidermal growth factor receptor (WJTOG3405): an open label, randomised phase 3 trial. *Lancet Oncol.* 2010;11(2):121–128.
13. Lee JS, Park K, Kim SW, et al. A randomized phase III study of gefitinib versus standard chemotherapy (gemcitabine plus cisplatin) as a first-line treatment for never-smokers with advanced or metastatic adenocarcinoma of the lung. *J Thorac Oncol.* 2009;4(9):S283.
14. Zhou C, Wu YL, et al. Efficacy results from the randomized phasae III OPTIMAL (CTONG 0802) study comparing first-line erlotinib versus carboplatin plus gemcitabine in Chinese advanced non-small cell lung cancer patients with EGFR activating mutations. *Annals of Oncology.* 2010;21(Supplement 8):viii6.
15. Yang CH, Fukuoka M, Mok TS, et al. Final overall survival (OS) results from a phase III, randomized, open-label, first-line study of gefitinib v. carboplatin/paclitaxel in clinically selected patients with advanced non-small cell lung cancer in ASIA (IPASS). *Annals of Oncology.* 2010;21(Supplement 8): viii1.

16. Pao W, Miller VA, Politi KA, et al. Acquired resistance of lung adenocarcinomas to gefitinib or erlotinib is associated with a second mutation in the EGFR kinase domain. PLoS Med. 2005 Mar;2(3):e73. Epub 2005 Feb 22.

17. Kobayashi S, Boggon TJ, Dayaram T, et al. EGFR mutation and resistance of non-small-cell lung cancer to gefitinib. *N Engl J Med.* 2005;352(8):786–792.

18. Oxnard GR, Arcila ME, Sima CS, et al. Acquired resistance to EGFR tyrosine kinase inhibitors in EGFR-mutant lung cancer: distinct natural history of patients with tumors harboring the T790M mutation. *Clin Cancer Res.* 2011;17(6):1616–1622.

19. Arcila ME, Oxnard GR, Nafa K, et al. Rebiopsy of lung cancer patients with acquired resistance to EGFR inhibitors and enhanced detection of the T790M mutation using a locked nucleic acid-based assay. *Clin Cancer Res.* 2011;17(5):1169–1180.

20. Karapetis, CS, Khambata-Ford S, Jonker DJ, et al. K-ras mutations and benefit from cetuximab in advanced colorectal cancer. *N Engl J Med.* 2008;359(17):1757–1765.

21. Horn L, Pao W. EML4-ALK: honing in on a new target in non-small-cell lung cancer. *J Clin Oncol.* 2009;27(26):4232–4235.

22. Shaw AT, Yeap BY, Mino-Kenudson M, et al. Clinical features and outcome of patients with non-small-cell lung cancer who harbor EML4-ALK. *J Clin Oncol.* 2009;27(26):4247–4253.

23. Kwak EL, Bang YJ, Camidge DR, et al. Anaplastic lymphoma kinase inhibition in non-small-cell lung cancer. *N Engl J Med.* 2010;363(18):1693–1703.

24. Sozzi G, Pastorino U, Moiraghi L, et al. Loss of FHIT function in lung cancer and preinvasive bronchial lesions. *Cancer Res.* 1998;58(22):5032–5037.

CHAPTER 4

Diagnosis and Staging of Lung Cancer

■ Signs and Symptoms of Lung Cancer

- The advent of CT screening for lung cancer will result in a rising incidence of the disease, and more patients diagnosed at earlier stages of disease before symptoms develop.

- Some patients with lung cancer have no symptoms, and their lung cancer is discovered incidentally on a CXR or CT scan performed for some other reason.

- Most people with lung cancer are diagnosed when their tumor grows to a size, or in a location, that causes symptoms.

- Symptoms of primary lung cancer include cough (which may or may not be associated with production of mucus or blood), shortness of breath, and/or chest pain.

- NSCLC may arise in the apex of the lung and invade upward beneath the clavicle, damaging the brachial plexus of nerves. This is called a lung cancer of the superior sulcus, or Pancoast tumor.
  - This results in shoulder pain as well as sensory and motor deficits in the ipsilateral arm, often in an ulnar nerve distribution.
  - Disruption of preganglionic sympathetic nerve fibers coursing near the apex of the lung may result in ipsilateral Horner's syndrome (pupillary miosis, eyelid ptosis, and facial anhidrosis).

- The most common sites of lung cancer metastasis are the lymph nodes, lung, bone, brain, liver, and adrenal glands. Common signs and/or symptoms due to lung cancer metastasis include:
  - Palpable lymphadenopathy in the neck or supraclavicular region
  - Bone pain
  - Abdominal pain

- Neurologic changes
- Headache
- Seizure

■ Lung cancer may generate fluid (i.e., malignant pleural effusion [MPE]) that accumulates in the chest and compresses the surrounding lung, which may result in rapidly progressive shortness of breath or chest discomfort.

■ Mediastinal tumors, or mediastinal lymph node metastases, which press on the superior vena cava and block blood return to the heart, may result in superior vena cava (SVC) syndrome.

- Physical signs include neck, facial, and/or bilateral arm swelling, with jugular venous distension and blooms of collateral blood vessels in the skin of the upper chest.

- Symptoms of SVC syndrome, such as facial or arm swelling, may be more noticeable to patients when they bend over or lie flat, or when they first get out of bed in the morning.

■ Hoarseness of the voice may occur in patients with lung cancer who have mediastinal invasion or mediastinal lymph node metastases, which injure the recurrent laryngeal nerve, resulting in unilateral vocal cord paralysis, typically on the left side.

■ Generalized symptoms, such as fatigue, malaise, and loss of appetite, are not necessarily due to metastases.

- Similar to when a patient has a viral illness, the presence of cancer in the body may release inflammatory cytokines, including tumor necrosis factor-alpha (TNF-a) and interleukin-6 (IL-6), which result in fatigue, anorexia, and weight loss even in patients with early-stage disease.

- Weight loss of 15% or more of the patient's baseline body weight during the previous 6 months is a poor prognostic factor.

■ Paraneoplastic syndromes related to lung cancer include changes in blood chemistry, such as low serum sodium (Na^+) or high blood calcium (Ca^{++}) levels, which can result in a variety of symptoms:

- Hyponatremia may result in nausea, anorexia, headache, restlessness, and/or confusion, or even seizure or coma.

* Hypercalcemia may result in arthralgias, myalgias, abdominal pain, cardiac arrhythmia, and polyuria with volume contraction, which can result in prerenal azotemia or acute renal failure.

■ Hypertrophic osteoarthropathy (HOA) is a paraneoplastic syndrome related to lung cancer that is characterized by periosteal new bone formation, bone pain, symmetric arthritis, and neurovascular changes, including erythema and paresthesias.

■ Clubbing of the fingernails is often associated with HOA or can occur independently in the setting of lung cancer.

■ Paraneoplastic syndromes resulting in neurologic problems are more common with SCLC and are rarely seen in patients with NSCLC.

  * Eaton-Lambert syndrome results from an immune response to the cancer that generates IgG antibodies against voltage-sensitive calcium channels at the neuromuscular junction of skeletal muscle.

    ■ Patients report easy fatiguability and generalized muscle weakness.

    ■ Physical signs include objective, symmetric muscle weakness, especially in the proximal arms and legs, with decreased deep tendon reflexes.

    ■ Muscle strength may improve with repeated muscle movement. This is the opposite of myasthenia gravis, in which muscle strength decreases with repeated movement.

  * Anti-Hu antibody syndrome is characterized by antibodies that destroy cerebral cortical neurons.

    ■ The most common symptom is sensory neuropathy. Motor dysfunction, memory loss, or dementia may also occur.

    ■ Damage to the autonomic nervous system may result in orthostatic hypotension and even cardiac arrhythmias.

    ■ Anti-Hu is one of several antibodies that may cause this syndrome. Other antigenic determinants are less well characterized.

  * Anti-Yo antibody syndrome is characterized by antibodies that destroy cerebellar neurons.

- Patients may present with ataxia, dysarthria, nystagmus, and difficulty with motor coordination.
- Neurologic findings are usually bilateral and symmetric.
- Cerebellar degeneration may also be associated with noncerebellar problems, including peripheral neuropathy and dementia.
  - Paraneoplastic neuropathy may be permanent, even if the underlying cancer is successfully treated.
  - Patients suspected of having autoimmune neuropathy should be evaluated by a neurologist, who may refer them for serologic tests, electromyography, and nerve conduction studies to confirm the diagnosis.

■ Diagnosis of Lung Cancer

- A biopsy is necessary to make the diagnosis of lung cancer.
- A diagnostic tissue sample may be obtained using several different strategies, which are listed below in rough order of increasing invasiveness and risk of morbidity to the patient:
  - Sputum cytology
  - Fine-needle aspiration
  - Thoracentesis
  - Core needle biopsy
  - Bronchoscopy
  - Mediastinoscopy
  - Thoracoscopy
  - Thoracotomy
- The physician should choose the target for biopsy based on physical examination and radiologic scans in order to establish the diagnosis and stage of disease in the safest and most efficient way possible.
- Given the need to distinguish squamous from non-squamous histology, the need to have adequate tissue for EGFR mutation testing, and ALK FISH, larger biopsies are needed for the management of patients with lung cancer.
- The goal of a biopsy should be to obtain more tissue than what can be obtained in a routine fine-needle aspirate.

- Multiple fine-needle aspirates can produce sufficient cells to create a cell pellet or cell block, which can then be encased in paraffin and ultimately analyzed for genetic changes.
- Core needle biopsy, or excisional biopsies, are preferred to provide the pathologist with sufficient tissue to examine tumor architecture and to have more tissue for molecular or immunohistochemical studies.

■ Staging of Non–Small Cell Lung Cancer

- The lungs have five lobes in all—three on the right (upper, middle, lower) and two on the left (upper, lower). Lymphatic drainage of the lungs is toward the center of the chest. Cancer cells that spread through the lymphatic system are often trapped and grow into tumors within hilar and mediastinal lymph nodes. **Figure 4.1** demonstrates the location of lung lobes and lymph nodes on a standard chest radiograph.
- Any patient with NSCLC who does not already have pathologic confirmation of metastatic disease should undergo a complete staging workup, including medical history and physical examination; laboratory analysis including complete blood count, electrolyte, and chemistry panel including liver function tests; and radiologic tests including CXR, CT that extends inferiorly to include the adrenal glands, and F-18-fluorodeoxyglucose positron emission tomography (FDG-PET) scan.

■ FDG-PET Scan

- Although no prospective, randomized study has been completed to demonstrate survival benefit for patients with lung cancer staged with FDG-PET scan, retrospective and nonrandomized data from patients with NSCLC confirm that, when added to CT scan, the information provided by FDG-PET significantly alters patient management.[1,2]
- FDG-PET scans have a high negative predictive value and corroborate negative CT scans to confirm early-stage NSCLC. In addition, FDG-PET scans identify unsus-

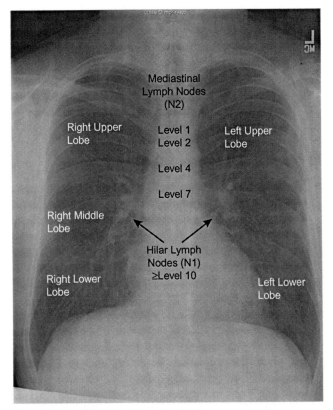

Figure 4.1 Anatomical considerations for lung cancer staging.

pected sites of metastasis, thereby redirecting biopsy and precluding unnecessary surgery or radiation in the face of metastatic disease.

■ In head-to-head testing, FDG-PET scans appear to be more sensitive than bone scans for detecting bone metastases.[3,4] However, not all FDG-PET scans include the long bones. Therefore, a radionuclide bone scan is indicated to detect bone metastasis in patients who might otherwise have early-stage disease, who have not already undergone an FDG-PET scan that included the long bones, and who are suspected of having bone metastasis due to bone pain or elevated blood calcium or alkaline phosphatase.

■ Imaging the Central Nervous System

■ For patients with lung cancer, magnetic resonance imaging (MRI) scans are commonly used to image the central nervous system. An MRI scan with gadolinium is the most sensitive test for detecting brain metastasis and is superior to CT scan of the brain with intravenous contrast for this purpose.[5]

■ MRI of the brain is indicated in patients with symptoms of brain metastasis (headache, neurologic changes, unexplained nausea) and is also commonly performed to screen patients with stage IB or greater NSCLC for occult metastasis before they commit to aggressive local therapy of their primary tumor, such as surgery or radiation.

■ MRI of the spine is useful to detect spine metastasis that has an epidural component or threatens spinal cord compression. Gadolinium enhancement of spine MRI is typically required to detect leptomeningeal metastasis.

■ Resectable Versus Unresectable NSCLC

■ The most practical way to think about NSCLC staging is to understand whether or not the cancer can be removed by a surgeon (i.e., is the tumor resectable, or is it unresectable?).

■ In general, stages I–II NSCLC tumors have a size, shape, and location that allow a surgeon to completely remove them.

- Stage I lung cancers are small in size (≤ 5 cm) and have not spread to any lymph nodes.
- Stage II lung cancers are either large in size (> 5 cm) or have spread to proximal lymph nodes (i.e., lymph nodes that are contained within the surrounding lung so that they may be removed in the same lobe(s) of lung, or along with the same bronchial branch of the lobe(s) where the cancer started).

■ Stage III NSCLC tumors are difficult, and sometimes impossible, to remove.

- When lung cancer spreads to the mediastinal lymph nodes (N2–3 nodes), the nodes are not included en bloc

with the resected lung specimen, and any lymph node
metastasis must be removed piecemeal with a procedure known as lymph node dissection.

- When the lung cancer has spread to mediastinal lymph
  nodes on the same side as where the cancer started
  (ipsilateral, N2), it is stage IIIA. Stage IIIA disease may
  still be considered resectable as long as the involved
  nodes are not bulky or too numerous.
- When the lung cancer has spread to lymph nodes on
  the opposite side of the chest (contralateral, N3) or in
  the supraclavicular region (N3), it is unresectable (stage
  IIIB).
- Other situations that make a stage III lung cancer impossible to remove are if the cancer invades vital structures within the chest (T4) (i.e., heart, large blood
  vessels, trachea).

- Lung cancers that have spread to different locations within
  the lobe of origin, so-called satellite nodules, are considered to be T3.
- Stage IV NSCLC has spread to the pleura or pericardium,
  often diagnosed by cancer cells found floating in pleural
  or pericardial fluid.
- Stage IV NSCLC more commonly spreads by way of the
  bloodstream to distant sites within the body, typically lung,
  liver, brain, adrenal, and bone.
- Stage IV NSCLC is not curable with surgery or radiation.
- The formal TNM staging criteria for NSCLC are presented
  in **Table 4.1**.

■ Staging of Small Cell Lung Cancer

- SCLC is prone to widespread, hematogenous metastasis
  so that very few patients with SCLC are treated with surgery, and almost all SCLC patients receive chemotherapy.
  Some patients with SCLC benefit from radiation therapy.
- The staging of SCLC (limited vs. extensive) helps identify
  which patients can be treated with external-beam radiation
  therapy (XRT) to the chest in addition to chemotherapy.
  - Limited stage means the cancer is located on one side
    of the chest, involving a single region of the lung and

Table 4.1A   Staging of Non-Small Cell Lung Cancer

Primary Tumor (T)	
TX	Primary tumor cannot be assessed, or tumor proven by the presence of malignant cells in sputum or bronchial washings but not visualized by imaging or bronchoscopy
T0	No evidence of primary tumor
Tis	Carcinoma *in situ*
T1	Tumor ≤ 3 cm in greatest dimension, surrounded by lung or visceral pleura, without bronchoscopic evidence of invasion more proximal than the lobar bronchus (i.e., not in the main bronchus) T1a Tumor ≤ 2 cm in greatest dimension T1b Tumor > 2 cm but ≤ 3 cm in greatest dimension
T2	Tumor > 3 cm but ≤ 7 cm or tumor with any of the following features (T2 tumors with these features are classified T2a if ≤ 5 cm) ▪ Involves main bronchus, ≥ 2 cm distal to the carina ▪ Invades the visceral pleura ▪ Associated with atelectasis or obstructive pneumonitis that extends to the hilar region but does not involve the entire lung
T2a T2b	Tumor > 3 cm but ≤ 5 cm in greatest dimension Tumor > 5 cm but ≤ 7 cm in greatest dimension
T3	Tumor > 7 cm, or one that directly invades any of the following: chest wall (including superior sulcus tumors), diaphragm, phrenic nerve, mediastinal pleura, parietal pericardium; or tumor in the main bronchus < 2 cm distal to the carina, but without involvement of the carina; or associated atelectasis or obstructive pneumonitis of the entire lung or separate tumor nodules(s) in the same lobe
T4	Tumor of any size that invades any of the following: mediastinum, heart, great vessels, trachea, recurrent laryngeal nerve, esophagus, vertebral body, carina; or separate tumor nodules in a different ipsilateral lobe
Regional Lymph Nodes (N)	
NX	Regional lymph nodes cannot be assessed
N0	No regional lymph node metastasis

Table 4.1A   continued

N1	Metastasis in ipsilateral peribronchial and/or ipsilateral hilar lymph nodes, and intrapulmonary nodes including involvement by direct extension of the primary tumor
N2	Metastasis in ipsilateral mediastinal and/or subcarinal lymph node(s)
N3	Metastasis in contralateral mediastinal, contralateral hilar, ipsilateral or contralateral scalene, or supraclavicular lymph node(s)

Distant Metastasis (M)

MX	Distant metastasis cannot be assessed
M0	No distant metastasis
M1	Distant metastasis
M1a	Separate tumor nodule(s) in a contralateral lobe; tumor with pleural nodules or malignant pleural or pericardial effusion
M1b	Distant metastases

Based on Goldstraw, Crowley J, Chansky K, et al. The IASLC Lung Cancer Staging Project: proposals for the revision of the TNM Stage Groupings in the forthcoming (seventh) edition of the TNM classification of malignant tumours. *J Thorac Oncol.* 2007;2(8):706–714.

adjacent lymph nodes, allowing the entire region to be treated with XRT. The minority of patients (40%) have limited-stage disease.

- Extensive stage means the cancer has spread to other regions of the chest, or outside of the chest, and cannot be treated with a single radiation field. Most patients (60%) have extensive-stage disease and are treated with chemotherapy only.

■ Any patient with SCLC who does not already have pathologic confirmation of extensive-stage disease should undergo a complete staging workup, including medical history and physical examination; laboratory analysis including complete blood count, electrolyte, and chemistry panel including liver function tests and LDH; and radiologic

Table 4.1B   Stage Groupings

Stage Groupings				5-Year Survival	
				Clinical Stage	Pathologic Stage
Occult Carcinoma	TX	N0	M0	-	-
0	Tis	N0	M0	-	-
IA	T1a,b	N0	M0	50%	73%
IB	T2a	N0	M0	43%	58%
IIA	T1a,b	N1	M0	36%	46%
	T2a	N1	M0		
	T2b	N0	M0		
IIB	T2b	N1	M0	25%	36%
	T3	N0	M0		
IIIA	T1,T2	N2	M0	19%	24%
	T3	N1,N2	M0		
	T4	N0,N1	M0		
IIIB	T4	N2	M0	7%	9%
	Any T	N3	M0		
IV	Any T	Any N	M1a,b	2%	13%

tests including CXR and CT that extends inferiorly to include the liver and adrenal glands, MRI or CT scan of the brain with contrast enhancement, and a radionuclide scan such as FDG-PET or bone scan.

- Due to the propensity of SCLC to spread to the brain, every patient with SCLC should undergo baseline MRI or CT scan of the brain with contrast enhancement, even in the absence of neurologic symptoms.

▪ At the conclusion of these tests, any patient who is presumed to have limited-stage disease but has unexplained elevation in his or her serum LDH or alkaline phosphatase should also undergo random unilateral or bilateral bone marrow biopsy of the posterior iliac crest to rule out occult bone metastasis.

▪ Clinical Stage Versus Pathologic Stage

▪ The results of history, physical examination, blood tests, and radiologic studies provide the physician with clinical evidence of the location and extent of the cancer. This is known as the clinical stage.

▪ The gold standard for staging lung cancer is to prove the presence of cancer with a biopsy. Only with a biopsy is the treating physician certain of the presence of cancer in a specific location.

▪ The biopsy-proven stage, or the stage established by pathologic analysis of the lung cancer after it is completely removed by a surgeon, is known as the pathologic stage.

▪ The preponderance of the clinical evidence may be sufficient to convince the treating physician of the patient's stage of disease.

  • For example, if a patient has back pain, CT scan or radiographic evidence of a lytic lesion in the spine, and abnormal uptake on bone scan or FDG-PET scan in the same location, the treating physician may be sufficiently convinced of clinical stage IV disease, metastatic to bone (M1), so as to avoid the morbidity of a bone biopsy.

  • However, whenever the clinical evidence is inconsistent or insufficient to establish the clinical stage, the treating physician must pursue biopsy to establish the pathologic stage before establishing the goals of therapy and embarking on treatment (see **Table 4.2**).

Table 4.2   Five-Year Survival of Lung Cancer Patients, Based on Stage

Non-Small Cell Lung Cancer		
Pathologic stage	2-year overall survival[1]	5-year overall survival[1]
IA	91%	73%
IB	80%	58%
IIA	71%	46%
IIB	58%	36%
IIIA	48%	24%
IIIB	22%	9%
IV	10%	1%

Small Cell Lung Cancer	
Clinical Stage	5-Year Survival
Limited Stage	16–26% [2]
Extensive Stage	0–10% [3]

Survival data adapted from:

[1]Goldstraw P, Crowley J, Chansky K, et al. The IASLC Lung Cancer Staging Project: proposals for the revision of the TNM stage groupings in the forthcoming (seventh) edition of the TNM Classification of malignant tumours. *J Thorac Oncol.* 2007;2:706–14.

[2]Turrisi AT, III, Kim K, Blum R, et al. Twice-daily compared with once-daily thoracic radiotherapy in limited small-cell lung cancer treated concurrently with cisplatin and etoposide. *N Engl J Med.* 1999;340:265–71.

[3]Noda K, Nishiwaki Y, Kawahara M, et al. Irinotecan plus cisplatin compared with etoposide plus cisplatin for extensive small-cell lung cancer. *N Engl J Med.* 2002;346:85–91.

■ References

1. Pfister DG, Johnson DH, Azzoli CG, et al. American Society of Clinical Oncology treatment of unresectable non-small-cell lung cancer guideline: update 2003. *J Clin Oncol.* 2004;22(2): 330–353.
2. Vansteenkiste J, Fischer BM, Dooms C, et al. Positron-emission tomography in prognostic and therapeutic assessment of lung cancer: systematic review. *Lancet Oncol.* 2004;5(9):531–540.
3. Bury T, Barreto A, Daenen F, et al. Fluorine-18 deoxyglucose positron emission tomography for the detection of bone metastases in patients with non-small cell lung cancer. *Eur J Nucl Med.* 1998;25(9):1244–1247.
4. Cheran SK, Herndon JE 2nd, Patz EF Jr. Comparison of whole-body FDG-PET to bone scan for detection of bone metastases in patients with a new diagnosis of lung cancer. *Lung Cancer.* 2004;44(3):317–325.
5. Yokoi K, Kamiya N, Matsuguma H, et al. Detection of brain metastasis in potentially operable non-small cell lung cancer: a comparison of CT and MRI. *Chest.* 1999;115(3):714–719.

CHAPTER 5

Treatment of Stage IV NSCLC

■ Chemotherapy for Stage IV NSCLC

- Stage IV NSCLC is not amenable to surgery or radiation therapy with curative intent.
- The goal of treatment in patients with stage IV disease is to control further growth or spread of the cancer for as long as possible, thereby prolonging life, while decreasing cancer-related symptoms. This approach is sometimes referred to as "palliative care."
- Systemic chemotherapy is the only treatment that has been proven to increase overall survival in patients with otherwise incurable NSCLC who have a good performance status.
  - Numerous clinical trials randomizing patients to chemotherapy or supportive care only have demonstrated this survival benefit.[1-4]
  - From a population standpoint, the benefits are small—about a 2-month improvement in median survival and improved control of cancer-related symptoms for patients with metastatic NSCLC.
  - However, on a patient-by-patient basis, effective chemotherapy means many months or even years of increased survival, and a better quality of life.
  - One way to communicate the potential benefit of chemotherapy to patients with stage IV NSCLC is to quote survival proportions at 1 year or at 2 years from the date of diagnosis.
    - With chemotherapy, patients are five times more likely to be alive at 1 year (proportion alive improves from 10% to 50%).

- With chemotherapy, patients are 10 times more likely to be alive at 2 years (proportion alive improves from 1% up to 10%) compared to supportive care only.
- The best way to improve immediate symptoms due to NSCLC is to shrink the cancer.
  - For the 10% of patients whose cancer contains an EGFR mutation, treatment with an oral inhibitor of the EGFR tyrosine kinase (gefitinib, erlotinib, or afatinib) has a high likelihood of shrinking the cancer, with response rates above 70%.
  - However, most patients with NSCLC do not have an EGFR mutation. For these patients, chemotherapy shrinks stage IV NSCLC substantially in less than 30% of patients.
  - Therefore, in patients less likely to respond to chemotherapy, the treating physician must first address any critical sites of metastasis before embarking on chemotherapy in order to more reliably palliate symptoms and ensure the patient is well enough to tolerate the side effects of chemotherapy.
  - **Table 5.1** lists several of these critical medical issues that must be addressed prior to chemotherapy in the majority of patients, and the necessary interventions.
- For all patients treated with chemotherapy, there is a point in their care when additional chemotherapy will be more harmful than helpful.
  - Similarly, in the absence of a molecular target that insures response to a targeted drug, there are no data to justify using chemotherapy in patients with metastatic lung cancer and poor performance status (Karnofsky Performance Status ≤ 50%, ECOG/Zubrod Performance Status ≥ 3). These patients should be treated with supportive care only.
  - The guiding principle for supportive care is to maximize patient comfort.
  - During chemotherapy, patients endure the ill effects of therapy with the goal of controlling their cancer.
  - During supportive care, any treatment, test, or procedure that would be difficult or uncomfortable for the patient to complete should be reconsidered.

Table 5.1   Clinical Problems and Interventions

Problem	Standard intervention
Symptomatic malignant pleural effusion	Chest tube thoracostomy and pleurodesis, thoracoscopic drainage, or ambulatory pleural catheter
Pericardial effusion with cardiac tamponade	Pericardial drain or surgical window
SVC Syndrome	Radiation therapy +/− anticoagulation
Obstructive pneumonia	Antibiotics, external beam radiation therapy
Empyema	Antibiotics, surgical debridement
Hemoptysis	Antibiotics, cough suppression, correction of coagulopathy, external beam radiation therapy
Symptomatic lung collapse	If endobronchial culprit lesion identified, bronchoscopy can be used to clear endobronchial tumor or stent insertion
Hypercalcemia	Bisphosphonate therapy, hydration
Hyponatremia (SIADH)	Free water restriction
Refractory pain from bone metastasis	Radiation therapy
Debilitating pathologic fracture, or impending fracture of weight-bearing bone	Orthopedic surgery
Symptomatic or threatening brain metastases	Surgery, radiosurgery, whole brain radiation
Symptomatic epidural metastases or spinal cord compression	External beam radiation therapy or surgery

- All patients with incurable, metastatic lung cancer should have a discussion with their physician in order to establish advanced directives, which are instructions for the physician in the event of critical illness or cardiopulmonary arrest.
- If a patient with incurable, metastatic lung cancer is sick enough to require artificial life support (intubation with mechanical ventilation), then his or her prognosis is grim.
- Patients with metastatic lung cancer who require artificial life support are subject to disease progression while on the ventilator and have little or no chance of coming off the ventilator.
- Such patients should not be subjected to the discomfort of cardiopulmonary resuscitation or artificial life support in the event of cardiopulmonary arrest. Instead, in the event of critical illness, comfort measures should be used to prevent pain and suffering at the end of life.
- Advanced directives are also known as "Do Not Resuscitate/Do Not Intubate" (DNR/DNI) orders.
- Each state has specific guidelines for patients and doctors to establish these orders and document them in the medical record.
- The cornerstone of a DNR/DNI order is a discussion among the patient, his or her healthcare proxy, and the attending physician in order to establish mutual understanding of the physician's advice and the patient's wishes.
- It is always best for this discussion to take place early in the course of treatment. However, if a patient does not have advanced directives in place, this discussion must take place as the patient is making the transition to supportive care only.
- The guiding principle of supportive care, namely, maximizing patient comfort, is perhaps best illustrated during a discussion of advance directives. Artificial life support is an extreme example of an inappropriate medical intervention for a patient with incurable metastatic lung cancer.

- Supportive care is not the same as end-of-life care. Lung cancer that is allowed to grow according to its natural history may take many months, or even years, to take a patient's life, especially if the cancer grows very slowly.

- Patients who are prescribed supportive care only should not feel that their oncologist has nothing to offer. On the contrary, there is always something that can be done to mitigate the symptoms of the cancer.

- Components of supportive care include, but are not limited to, antibiotics, pain medication, supplemental oxygen, bronchodilators, corticosteroids, antitussive agents, antiemetics, appetite stimulants, blood transfusions, physical and occupational therapy, psychosocial support or psychiatric care, and home nursing care and support.

- End-of-life care is often referred to as hospice care.

- Patients at the end of life often take to bed in their final days due to the their cancer symptoms.

- Patients who are limited to bed may be difficult to care for at home. These patients are often better served in an inpatient facility that provides 24-hour nursing care for the dying patient.

- Most hospice organizations also provide home hospice services. During home hospice care, nurses and doctors come to the house to provide support for the dying patient and his or her family. However, the family provides the bulk of the nursing care.

- In addition to a focus on comfort and quality of life, palliative care includes emotional and psychological support and education of patients and their families regarding death and dying.

- A prospective trial designed to measure the impact of regimented palliative care on the outcome of patients with stage IV NSCLC enrolled 151 patients and randomized them to standard oncologic care versus standard oncologic care plus early palliative care, which included focus on symptom control and psychosocial support.[5]

  - Patients were educated about death and dying and the importance of establishing advance directives to

Patient must have pathologically confirmed stage IV; histologic sample preferred to distinguish squamous from non-squamous histology, and for molecular testing. No critical metastases. Karnofsky performance status ≥60% (ECOG ≤2). When selecting chemotherapy, always consider enrolling the patient in a clinical trial. It is reasonable to delay cytotoxic chemotherapy to await molecular test results if the pace of the disease allows, and no anticipated deterioration of performance status.

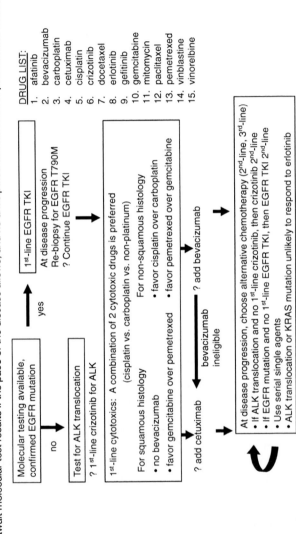

DRUG LIST:
1. afatinib
2. bevacizumab
3. carboplatin
4. cetuximab
5. cisplatin
6. crizotinib
7. docetaxel
8. erlotinib
9. gefitinib
10. gemcitabine
11. mitomycin
12. paclitaxel
13. pemetrexed
14. vinblastine
15. vinorelbine

Molecular testing available, confirmed EGFR mutation

no

yes → 1st-line EGFR TKI

At disease progression
Re-biopsy for EGFR T790M
? Continue EGFR TKI

Test for ALK translocation
? 1st-line crizotinib for ALK

1st-line cytotoxics: A combination of 2 cytotoxic drugs is preferred
(cisplatin vs. carboplatin vs. non-platinum)

For squamous histology
• no bevacizumab
• favor gemcitabine over pemetrexed

For non-squamous histology
• favor cisplatin over carboplatin
• favor pemetrexed over gemcitabine

? add bevacizumab

bevacizumab ineligible

? add cetuximab

At disease progression, choose alternative chemotherapy (2nd-line, 3rd-line)
• If ALK translocation and no 1st-line crizotinib, then crizotinib 2nd-line
• If EGFR mutation and no 1st-line EGFR TKI, then EGFR TKI 2nd-line
• Use serial single agents
• ALK translocation or KRAS mutation unlikely to respond to erlotinib

Figure 5.1 Selection of chemotherapy for stage IV NSCLC.

prevent futile medical interventions in the face of progressive incurable cancer and life-threatening illness.

* Patients randomized to early palliative care had lower rates of depression, better quality of life, better mood, and received less aggressive care at the end of life.

* Despite the lack of aggressive care at the end of life, patients randomized to early palliative care lived longer than patients who received only standard oncologic care (median survival 11.6 vs. 8.9 months, P = 0.02).[5]

■ Chemotherapy also improves survival, and proper selection of chemotherapy improves the patient's chances of clinical benefit.

■ A working algorithm for selection of chemotherapy for patients with stage IV NSCLC, based on clinical trial data which are discussed in this chapter, is presented and summarized in **Figure 5.1**.

■ Clinical Trials

■ Better treatments for metastatic lung cancer are sorely needed. The development of all the chemotherapy drugs discussed in this chapter, and the treatments of the future, are dependent upon patient participation in clinical research.

■ Given the poor outcomes of patients with metastatic lung cancer and the limitations of current therapy, it is reasonable for a patient with incurable metastatic NSCLC to enroll in a clinical trial of novel chemotherapy at any time in the course of his or her treatment, including first-line chemotherapy.

■ Patients who participate in clinical trials are among the first to receive new chemotherapy drugs. However, there is no guarantee that the new treatment will be safe, effective, or better than a standard treatment.

■ In order to join a clinical trial, patients must complete a learning process known as informed consent.

* During informed consent, the physician must list all of the patient's options, so that the person understands the standard treatments and how the new treatment differs.

- The physician must also list all of the risks of the new treatment, which may or may not be different from the risks of standard treatment.
- Finally, the physician must explain what will be required of each patient in order to participate in the clinical trial, including the number of doctor visits, specific tests, and the schedule of treatment.
- If the physician feels the patient understands all of the potential risks and benefits of participating in a clinical trial and the patient decides to participate, then both the patient and the physician sign an informed consent document, which is a record of their mutual understanding.
- Even after the patient and physician sign the informed consent document, the learning process continues. The patient should be aware that he or she may withdraw from a clinical trial at any time.
- Clinical trials are often described as being in phase 1, 2, or 3.
  - The goal of a phase 1 clinical trial is to prove that a new drug or treatment that has proven to be safe for use in animals may also be given safely to humans. Patients who participate in phase 1 clinical trials are often the first human beings ever to receive a new chemotherapy drug.
  - Once a new drug or treatment has been proven to be safe to give to humans and the proper dose has been chosen in a phase 1 clinical trial, the same drug, dose, and schedule is then studied in a phase 2 clinical trial. Phase 2 clinical trials are designed to prove that a new drug or treatment is effective in treating cancer. Common measures of efficacy include radiologic response rate (RR), symptom improvement, time to progression (TTP), and overall survival (OS).
  - Phase 3 clinical trials are designed to show that a new treatment is better than a standard treatment.
    - Phase 3 trials often require patients to be randomized between a new treatment and a standard treatment.
    - In order to control for the placebo effect (i.e., the natural tendency of patients to feel better if they

are given any treatment), patients randomized to the control arm of a phase 3 clinical trial are often given a placebo so that they are not aware of whether they are receiving additional therapy.

* Randomization is often distressing to patients, who do not want their treatment determined by the flip of a coin. However, if the phase 3 clinical trial is well designed, it should not matter to the patient or the physician to which treatment the patient is assigned, because both treatments are potentially effective.

■ First-Line Chemotherapy

* Any patient with metastatic NSCLC, adequate performance status (≥ 70% on the Karnofsky performance scale [KPS] or ECOG/Zubrod ≤ 2), and no critical sites of metastasis should be offered chemotherapy. The ECOG/Zubrod and KPS are detailed in **Table 5.2**.

* For patients with NSCLC and EGFR mutation, the chance of clinical benefit from treatment with an EGFR tyrosine kinase inhibitor is so high, and the chance of harm is so low, that these patients should be offered treatment with drugs like gefitinib, erlotinib, or afatinib even if they have a poor performance status.

* Clinical trials are underway to discover if targeted tyrosine kinase inhibitors are more effective than other drugs for patients with EML4-ALK translocation. The first drug being tested in randomized trials in this regard is the ALK inhibitor crizotinib (Xalkori).

* The final decision about which chemotherapy to use first should be made by the treating medical oncologist, taking into account molecular and histologic characteristics of the patient's cancer, the results of randomized clinical trials, side effect profiles of the drugs, and patient preferences regarding side effects and schedule.

* Even with advances in treatment selection based on molecular and histologic characteristics, the current determining factor in prescribing chemotherapy for metastatic NSCLC remains "trial and error."

Table 5.2   Scales of Performance Status

Zubrod performance scale		Karnofsky performance scale	
0	Normal activity. Able to carry on normal activity and to work. No special care is needed.	100%	Normal; no complaints; no evidence of disease.
1	Symptoms, but nearly fully ambulatory.	90%	Able to carry on normal activity; minor signs or symptoms of disease.
		80%	Normal activity with effort; some signs or symptoms of disease.
2	Some bed time, but needs to be in bed less than 50% of normal daytime. Unable to work. Able to live at home, care for most personal needs. A varying amount of assistance is needed.	70%	Cares for self. Unable to carry on normal activity or to do active work.
		60%	Requires occasional assistance, but is able to care for most of his/her needs.
3	Needs to be in bed more than 50% of normal daytime.	50%	Requires considerable assistance and frequent medical care. Unable to care for self. Requires equivalent of institutional or hospital care. Disease may be progressing rapidly.
		40%	Disabled; requires special care and assistance.
4	Unable to get out of bed.	30%	Severely disabled; hospitalization is indicated although death not imminent.

Table 5.2   continued

Zubrod performance scale		Karnofsky performance scale	
4		20%	Very sick; hospitalization necessary; active supportive treatment necessary.
		10%	Moribund; fatal processes progressing rapidly.
		0%	Dead

Adapted from Orr ST, Aisner J. Performance status assessment among oncology patients: a review. *Cancer Treat Rep.* 1986;70:1423–9.

- The treating oncologist chooses what he or she thinks is the best chemotherapy regimen to try first.
- If the cancer grows despite treatment, alternative drugs may be considered in turn (see **Table 5.3**).

▪ For patients whose EGFR mutation status is negative or unknown, combination chemotherapy using the cytotoxic drug cisplatin (Platinol), combined with another drug, is the gold standard treatment for patients with metastatic NSCLC. This superiority is based on both convention and the preponderance of clinical trial evidence.

- Cisplatin is a metal salt that causes DNA strand breaks, leading to programmed cell death (apoptosis).
- Cisplatin is challenging to deliver, with potential side effects including nausea, vomiting, peripheral nerve damage, kidney damage, and hearing loss.
- Cisplatin must be administered with high volumes of intravenous fluid to maintain urine output to protect the kidneys. Patients are also encouraged to increase their oral intake of fluids the day before and the day after administration of cisplatin to maintain their urine output at home. This may be difficult if the patient experiences nausea or vomiting.

Table 5.3   Selected Commonly Used Chemotherapy Regimens for the Treatment of Patients with Stage IV NSCLC

Regimen	Reference
Pemetrexed 500 mg/m² IV on day 1 Cisplatin 75 mg/m2 IV on day 1 Repeat every 21 days	1
Pemetrexed 500 mg/m² IV on day 1 Carboplatin AUC = 5 IV on day 1 Repeat every 21 days	2
Paclitaxel 175–225 mg/m² IV over 3 hours on day 1 Carboplatin AUC = 6 IV on day 1 Repeat every 21 days	3
Docetaxel 75 mg/m² IV over 60 min on day 1 Carboplatin AUC = 6 IV on day 1 Repeat every 21 days	4
Docetaxel 75 mg/m² IV over 60 min day 1 Cisplatin 75 mg/m² IV day 1 Repeat every 21 days	4
Gemcitabine 1000–1200 mg/m² IV days 1 and 8 Carboplatin AUC = 5 IV on day 1 (or day 8) Repeat every 21 days	5,6,7
Gemcitabine 1000 mg/m² IV days 1, 8, (15) Cisplatin 80–100 mg/m² IV on day 8 or 15 Repeat every 21–28 days	3,6,7
Mitomycin 8 mg/m² IV push on days 1, 29, and 71 (limit 3 doses of mitomycin) Vinblastine 4 mg/m² IV push on day 1; then Vinblastine 2 mg/m² on day 8; then Vinblastine 4.5 mg/m² days 15, 22, 29, and every 2 weeks thereafter Cisplatin 100 mg/m² IVPB over 60 min days 1, 29, and every 6 weeks thereafter	8,9
Docetaxel 75 mg/m² IV over 60 min. Repeat every 21 days.	10
Docetaxel 35 mg/m² IV over 30 min weekly for up to 6 weeks in a row, 1–2 week break before recycling	11
Gemcitabine 1000 mg/m² IV over 30 min days 1, 8, (15) Repeat every 21–28 days	12

Table 5.3 continued

Regimen	Reference
Vinorelbine 30 mg/m² IV on days 1, 8 Repeat every 21 days	13
Erlotinib 150 mg (flat dose) by mouth daily	14
Pemetrexed 500 mg/m² IV over 10 min. Repeat every 21 days	15
According to NCCN guidelines, bevacizumab or cetuximab can be added to a variety of cytotoxic chemotherapies for selected patients as follows:	
+ Bevacizumab 15 mg/kg IV on day 1 Repeat every 21 days	16
+ Cetuximab 500 mg/m² IV on day 1, then 250 mg/m² on day 8 and weekly thereafter Repeat weekly	17

1. Scagliotti GV, Parikh P, von Pawel J, et al. Phase III study comparing cisplatin plus gemcitabine with cisplatin plus pemetrexed in chemotherapy-naive patients with advanced-stage non-small-cell lung cancer. *J Clin Oncol.* 2008;26:3543–51.

2. Gronberg BH, Bremnes RM, Flotten O, et al. Phase III study by the Norwegian lung cancer study group: pemetrexed plus carboplatin compared with gemcitabine plus carboplatin as first-line chemo-therapy in advanced non-small-cell lung cancer. *J Clin Oncol.* 2009;27:3217–24.

3. Schiller JH, Harrington D, Belani CP, et al. Comparison of four chemotherapy regimens for advanced non-small-cell lung cancer. *N Engl J Med.* 2002; 346:92–8.

4. Fossella F, Pereira JR, von Pawel J, et al. Randomized, multinational, phase III study of docetaxel plus platinum combinations versus vinorelbine plus cisplatin for advanced non-small-cell lung cancer: the TAX 326 study group. *J Clin Oncol.* 2003;21:3016–24.

5. Zatloukal P, Petruzelka L, Zemanova M, et al. Gemcitabine plus cisplatin vs. gemcitabine plus carboplatin in stage IIIb and IV non-small cell lung cancer: a phase III randomized trial. *Lung Cancer.* 2003;41:321–31.

6. Abratt RP, Sandler A, Crino L, et al. Combined cisplatin and gemcitabine for non-small cell lung cancer: influence of scheduling on toxicity and drug delivery. *Semin Oncol.* 1998;25:35–43.

Table 5.3 continued

7. Ricci S, Antonuzzo A, Galli L, et al. A randomized study comparing two different schedules of administration of cisplatin in combination with gemcitabine in advanced nonsmall cell lung carcinoma. *Cancer.* 2000;89:1714–9.

8. Danson S, Middleton MR, O'Byrne KJ, et al. Phase III trial of gemcitabine and carboplatin versus mitomycin, ifosfamide, and cisplatin or mitomycin, vinblastine, and cisplatin in patients with advanced nonsmall cell lung carcinoma. *Cancer.* 2003;98:542–53.

9. Gralla RJ, Kris MG, Potanovich LM, et al. Enhancing the Safety and Efficacy of the MVP Regimen (Mitomycin+Vinblastine+Cisplatin) in 100 Patients with Inoperable Non-small Cell Lung Cancer (NSCLC). *Proc Am Soc Clin Oncol.* [Abstract 888] 1989; 8:227.

10. Fossella FV, DeVore R, Kerr RN, et al. Randomized phase III trial of docetaxel versus vinorelbine or ifosfamide in patients with advanced non-small-cell lung cancer previously treated with platinum-containing chemotherapy regimens. The TAX 320 Non-Small Cell Lung Cancer Study Group. *J Clin Oncol.* 2000;18:2354–62.

11. Hainsworth JD, Burris HA, 3rd, Litchy S, et al. Weekly docetaxel in the treatment of elderly patients with advanced nonsmall cell lung carcinoma. A Minnie Pearl Cancer Research Network Phase II Trial. *Cancer.* 2000;89:328–33.

12. ten Bokkel Huinink WW, Bergman B, Chemaissani A, et al. Single-agent gemcitabine: an active and better tolerated alternative to standard cisplatin-based chemotherapy in locally advanced or metastatic non-small cell lung cancer. *Lung Cancer.* 1999;26:85–94.

13. Gridelli C, Perrone F, Gallo C, et al. Chemotherapy for elderly patients with advanced non-small-cell lung cancer: the Multicenter Italian Lung Cancer in the Elderly Study (MILES) phase III randomized trial. *J Natl Cancer Inst.* 2003;95:362–72.

14. Shepherd FA, Rodrigues Pereira J, Ciuleanu T, et al. Erlotinib in previously treated non-small-cell lung cancer. *N Engl J Med.* 2005;353:123–32.

15. Hanna N, Shepherd FA, Fossella FV, et al. Randomized phase III trial of pemetrexed versus docetaxel in patients with non-small-cell lung cancer previously treated with chemotherapy. *J Clin Oncol.* 2004;22:1589–97.

16. Sandler A, Gray R, Perry MC, et al. Paclitaxel-carboplatin alone or with bevacizumab for non-small-cell lung cancer. *N Engl J Med.* 2006;355:2542–50.

17. Pirker R, Pereira JR, Szczesna A, et al. Cetuximab plus chemotherapy in patients with advanced non-small-cell lung cancer (FLEX): an open-label randomised phase III trial. *Lancet.* 2009;373:1525–31.

- Antiemetic medications—including corticosteroids; serotonin receptor antagonists (ondansetron [Zofran] granisetron [Kytril], dolasetron [Anzemet], palonosetron [Aloxi]; and the neurokinin-1 receptor antagonist aprepitant (Emend)—should be used to prevent acute and delayed nausea and vomiting.[6,7]

■ Given the challenges of administering cisplatin, a related drug, carboplatin (Paraplatin), has been substituted for cisplatin for the treatment of NSCLC. Carboplatin is less likely to cause nausea or damage kidneys or peripheral nerves and is delivered without the need for additional intravenous fluid.

- There is debate as to whether combination chemotherapy using carboplatin is as effective as cisplatin combinations, and some data suggest that cisplatin is superior to carboplatin, especially because cisplatin combinations have a higher response rate.[8]

- A meta-analysis of all clinical trials comparing cisplatin with carboplatin and involving more than 2900 patients has shown that cisplatin combinations have a higher response rate, and there is a 10% reduction in the risk of death when using cisplatin compared to carboplatin when combined with modern chemotherapy drugs such as vinorelbine, gemcitabine, and taxanes.[9]

- The benefit in overall survival is so small and the potential increase in toxicity is so large that most published treatment guidelines suggest that carboplatin and cisplatin are equally acceptable for the treatment of patients with incurable, metastatic disease.[10–12]

- For patients without contraindication to cisplatin and in whom shrinking the cancer may offer symptom improvement, cisplatin is favored over carboplatin because of its higher response rate.

■ Phase 3 clinical trial data suggest that a platinum drug (cisplatin or carboplatin) should be combined with one other cytotoxic drug with a different mechanism of action that is synergistic with cisplatin effect.

■ Cytotoxic drugs to combine with cisplatin or carboplatin:

- Docetaxel (Taxotere) is a semi-synthetic taxane. Its mechanism of action is to bind to tubulin and inhibit cellular mitosis. Its dose-limiting toxicity is neutropenia, and common side effects include hair loss, diarrhea, mucositis, hypersensitivity, and neuropathy.

* Gemcitabine (Gemzar) is a fluorinated analog of cytosine that blocks enzymes necessary for DNA replication and also results in chain termination, followed by programmed cell death. Common side effects include lowering of the blood counts (neutropenia, thrombocytopenia, anemia) and peripheral edema, but it does not cause hair loss.
* Irinotecan (Camptosar) is a topoisomerase inhibitor that interferes with DNA replication followed by programmed cell death. It is unpopular in North America due to common gastrointestinal side effects including diarrhea and stomach upset, as well as cytopenias.
* Paclitaxel (Taxol) is a taxane that also binds to tubulin to block cellular mitosis. Its dose-limiting toxicity is neutropenia. It also causes hair loss and peripheral neuropathy, and is associated with hypersensitivity due to the solvent (Cremaphor) in which it is dissolved in order to be administered IV.
* Albumin-bound paclitaxel (Abraxane) has a similar mechanism of action to paclitaxel and is not associated with infusion reactions because the drug is suspended in solution by albumin. This packaging of the drug may also enhance cytotoxicity, with potential for enhanced cytotoxicity against squamous NSCLC.
* Pemetrexed (Alimta) is a multitargeted antifolate drug that primarily blocks the enzyme thymidylate synthase (TS) to prevent nucleoside formation necessary for DNA synthesis. It also blocks the enzymes DHFR and GARFT. Pemetrexed is most effective againse nonsquamous tumors, which may be due in part to lower expression of TS in these tumors.
* Vinorelbine (Navelbine) is a vinca alkaloid that binds to tubulin and inhibits cellular mitosis. The main side effects include neutropenia, peripheral neuropathy, abdominal cramps or constipation, and irritation of peripheral veins due to the drug's vesicant properties. Rare

infusion reactions have occurred, causing pain in the tumor, myalgias, or arthralgias.

■ A phase 3 clinical trial randomized more than 1200 patients with stage IV NSCLC to one of four modern, platinum-based chemotherapy regimens: cisplatin plus paclitaxel, cisplatin plus docetaxel, cisplatin plus gemcitabine, or carboplatin plus paclitaxel.[10] The results of this trial showed that RRs and OS were equivalent in all four treatment arms.

■ Nonplatinum combinations (gemcitabine plus paclitaxel, gemcitabine plus docetaxel) have been shown to be as effective as platinum-containing combinations but are not less toxic, having similar levels of cytopenia and asthenia.[13,14]

■ Two-drug combinations are more effective than single-agent therapy in terms of both RR and OS in head-to-head trials with patients with a good performance status.[15–17]

■ Patients treated with two-drug combination chemotherapy have an RR of about 20% to 30%. In other words, there is a 20% to 30% chance that their cancer will shrink in size by 50% or more.

■ The median survival of patients with metastatic NSCLC treated with combination chemotherapy is about 11 months.[18]

■ There is a significant risk of chemotherapy-related death (3–5% of all patients), most commonly due to lethal infections that occur during periods of neutropenia. Patients should be made aware of this risk of death and told to take any symptoms of infection or postchemotherapy fevers very seriously.

■ Most two-drug combinations for the treatment of metastatic NSCLC are relatively equivalent in terms of efficacy (RR and OS). However, there are important differences between certain two-drug cytotoxic chemotherapy regimens in terms of efficacy and side effects. For example:

  • Using carboplatin instead of cisplatin lowers the chance of radiologic response and may slightly lower efficacy in terms of overall survival. Compared to cisplatin, carboplatin reduces the risk of nausea, vomiting, peripheral neuropathy, hearing loss, and kidney damage but may result in higher rates of cytopenias, including leukopenia, anemia, and thrombocytopenia.[10]

- The combination of carboplatin plus paclitaxel is less likely to cause nausea or thrombocytopenia but results in hair loss and may cause peripheral neuropathy (numbness, tingling, and/or paresthesias in the fingers and toes), which may or may not be permanent.[11]

- The combination of carboplatin plus docetaxel is less likely to cause neuropathy than carboplatin plus paclitaxel but is more likely to result in cytopenias, including neutropenia with fever.[8]

- Carboplatin plus gemcitabine does not cause hair loss or neuropathy but results in higher rates of cytopenia than carboplatin plus paclitaxel and requires an extra day of treatment during each treatment cycle.

- A randomized trial of cisplatin plus docetaxel versus cisplatin plus vinorelbine showed that cisplatin plus docetaxel was slightly superior in efficacy in an unselected population of patients with stage IV NSCLC.[8]

- A large randomized trial that compared cisplatin plus pemetrexed versus cisplatin plus gemcitabine showed that cisplatin plus pemetrexed was superior in efficacy to cisplatin plus gemcitabine in subgroups of patients with nonsquamous histology. As a result, pemetrexed is only FDA approved for the treatment of patients with nonsquamous histology, and gemcitabine has fallen out of favor for first-line use in nonsquamous populations.[18]

■ Neutrophil and Red Blood Growth Factor Support

- Anemia and neutropenia due to chemotherapy can be reversed with synthetic growth factors that stimulate red blood cell and neutrophil production from the bone marrow.

- Synthetic cytokines have never been shown to improve the outcome of patients with lung cancer—namely, the RR to chemotherapy or OS.

- Filgrastim (Neupogen), and longer-acting pegylated preparations (Neulasta), are effective in reducing the duration of neutropenia following chemotherapy, thereby decreasing length of hospitalization.[19]
  - Filgrastim may be used to shorten white blood cell nadir in patients with fever or active infection following cytotoxic chemotherapy.
  - In patients who have experienced febrile neutropenia or dangerous infections following initial chemotherapy, it is reasonable to use prophylactic filgrastim to minimize the risk of febrile neutropenia in subsequent cycles of chemotherapy.
  - Alternatives to prophylactic filgrastim include lowering the dose of chemotherapy in subsequent cycles or lengthening the interval between treatments to allow more time for bone marrow recovery.
- Synthetic stimulants of red blood cell growth, such as erythropoietin alfa (Epogen, Procrit, or darbepoetin alfa [Aranesp]), can be used to treat fatigue in the setting of chemotherapy-induced anemia (serum hemoglobin $< 10\,g/dL$).[20]
  - Patients with anemia should be evaluated for blood loss prior to administration of erythropoietin.
  - Red blood cell transfusion, an alternative to erythropoietin treatment in lung cancer patients, is preferred in cases of severe anemia.
- Clinical trials of erythrocyte-stimulating agents in patients with lung cancer that attempted to raise serum hemoglobin to normal levels (i.e., from $12\,g/dL$ up to $15\,g/dL$) showed an increase in the risk of death. Patients must be informed of this potential increased risk of death in these trials prior to being treated with erythrocyte-stimulating agents.[20]

■ Targeted and Biological Chemotherapy

- Angiogenesis inhibitors:
  - Bevacizumab (Avastin) is a monoclonal antibody that binds to and deactivates a protein called vascular endothelial growth factor (VEGF), which would otherwise

promote new blood vessel formation that tumors require to grow.

* Results of a phase 3 clinical trial adding bevacizumab to carboplatin plus paclitaxel in patients with previously untreated, stage IV, nonsquamous NSCLC demonstrates that the addition of bevacizumab improves OS, progression-free survival (PFS), and objective response rate (ORR) compared with carboplatin plus paclitaxel alone.[21]

* Patients with squamous cell carcinoma were excluded from this study due to life-threatening and fatal pulmonary bleeding observed during phase 2 testing of the carboplatin plus paclitaxel plus bevacizumab combination in this histologic subtype. Patients with brain metastasis or those requiring anticoagulation for venous thromboembolic disease were also excluded due to the perceived risk of bleeding following treatment with bevacizumab.

* Despite exclusion of these high-risk patients, 1% of patients treated with bevacizumab on this study died of treatment-related hemoptysis, and there was also an increased risk of febrile neutropenia.

* In an elderly population, the increased risk of death related to febrile neutropenia caused by bevacizumab was such that no survival benefit was seen in this population.[22]

* A companion study that added bevacizumab to the cytotoxic drug combination cisplatin plus gemcitabine showed similar improvement in ORR and PFS. Perhaps due to the unexpectedly good survival in the control arm of 13 months, this trial failed to show a benefit to OS.[23]

* This study also showed similar efficacy whether bevacizumab was delivered at a high dose (15 mg/kg IV every 3 weeks) versus low dose (7.5 mg/kg IV every 3 weeks).

* In summary, bevacizumab improves OS when combined with carboplatin plus paclitaxel in nonsquamous patients and improves ORR and PFS when combined with a variety of chemotherapy regimens.

- As a result, bevacizumab is perhaps most useful for patients with symptomatic NSCLC (shortness of breath, cough, bone pain) in whom shrinking the cancer is important to improve quality of life.
- EGFR inhibitors:
  - The utility of epidermal growth factor receptor (EGFR) tyrosine kinase inhibitors in patients with EGFR mutation is well established.
  - Five prospective randomized trials in patients with metastatic, EGFR mutant NSCLC have shown that gefitinib or erlotinib provide these patients with higher rates of radiologic response and longer progression-free intervals compared to cytotoxic chemotherapy.[24–29]
  - Patients with an EGFR mutation detected in their lung cancer should receive first-line chemotherapy with gefitinib, erlotinib, or afatinib because of improved response rate, progression-free interval, and improved quality of life compared to traditional cytotoxic chemotherapy.
  - Patients who have an EGFR mutation discovered during first-line cytotoxic chemotherapy should be considered for switch maintenance, or early second-line use of an EGFR tyrosine kinase inhibitor.
  - Another drug that targets EGFR is cetuximab (Erbitux), which is a monoclonal antibody designed to bind to the extracellular domain of the EGFR protein.
  - A phase 3 trial enrolled patients with detectable EGFR expression by immunohistochemistry to standard cisplatin-based combination chemotherapy versus chemotherapy plus cetuximab.[30]
  - The results of this study showed that cetuximab improves overall survival. However, the magnitude of the benefit is less than that seen with the addition of bevacizumab to carboplatin plus paclitaxel.
  - Subgroup analyses failed to show that the benefit of cetuximab is higher in K-ras wildtype patients (a phenomenon observed in patients with metastatic colorectal cancer).[31]

- Other subgroup analyses have tried to distill the benefit of cetuximab based on other factors. For example, patients who develop skin rash during cycle 1 of cetuximab treatment garner more survival benefit. In addition, patients whose tumors express higher levels of EGFR protein, as measured by immunohistochemistry, garner more survival benefit.[32,33]
- Prospective trials to validate and further explore these observations are planned.

- ALK inhibitors:
  - ALK is a proto-oncogene growth kinase in the cytoplasm of cancer cells that becomes overactive due to translocations resulting in fusion genes.
  - Compared with non-ALK patients, patients with EML4-ALK mutant tumors tend to be younger, more likely to be men, more likely to be never or former light smokers, and tend to have adenocarcinomas (predominantly signet ring subtype).[34]
  - Patients with EML4-ALK translocation are resistant to EGFR tyrosine kinase inhibitors.[34]
  - A novel tyrosine kinase inhibitor specific to ALK (crizotinib [Xalkori]) has shown promising activity in patients with metastatic NSCLC and ALK translocation in a phase 1 clinical trial. In 2011, crizotinib was approved by the FDA as treatment for patients with stage IV NSCLC and ALK translocation based on the results of two phase 2 studies.[35]
  - Like EGFR mutation testing, the need for routine testing of NSCLC for ALK translocation in order to select optimal chemotherapy is now a standard of care.
  - ALK can be detected in NSCLC tumor tissue using fluorescent in situ hybridization (FISH), with PCR and immunohistochemical tests also in development.

■ Chemotherapy in the Elderly and Patients with Poor Performance Status

- Performance status is a more important predictor of treatment benefit than age.

- Age has never been shown to predict benefit from chemotherapy in NSCLC trials; however, older patients are more likely to experience dose-limiting or life-threatening side effects.
- Elderly patients with good performance status and no comorbid illness may be offered combination chemotherapy.
  - A randomized trial in elderly patients showed a significant improvement in overall survival for elderly patients treated with combination chemotherapy instead of single-agent chemotherapy.[36]
  - A subgroup analysis of a randomized trial comparing single-agent with combination chemotherapy demonstrated longer survival with combination chemotherapy, even in patients older than 70 years of age.[37]
- Elderly patients with poor fitness (KPS < 70%, ECOG/Zubrod ≥ 2) or significant comorbid illness should be treated with single-agent chemotherapy or best supportive care.
- Although two drugs are better than one in terms of RR and OS, single-agent chemotherapy causes fewer side effects than combination chemotherapy, with less likelihood of causing life-threatening neutropenia.
- Single-agent vinorelbine, docetaxel, and paclitaxel have each been shown to improve survival in previously untreated patients over best supportive care.[38–40]
- Single-agent chemotherapy may be appropriate for patients with comorbid illnesses that preclude risking the added side effects of combination chemotherapy.
- Single-agent chemotherapy is also appropriate for patients with poor performance status (KPS 60–70%, ECOG/Zubrod = 2).

■ Chemotherapy Guided by Pathologic or Molecular Characteristics of NSCLC

- To summarize the information presented earlier in this chapter, NSCLC is currently subdivided into the following clinically important subgroups:
  - Patients whose cancer harbors an EGFR mutation should receive first-line chemotherapy with an oral

EGFR tyrosine kinase inhibitor (gefitinib, erlotinib, or afatinib).

- Patients whose cancer harbors an ALK translocation should receive crizotinib, and a clinical trial to establish its utility as a first-line therapy is underway.
- Fit patients whose cancer has been tested and found not to harbor an EGFR mutation or have a K-ras mutation should not receive first-line EGFR tyrosine kinase inhibitor. Instead, these patients should be treated with first-line platinum-based combination chemotherapy.
- Patients whose cancer has squamous histology should not receive the drugs pemetrexed or bevacizumab.
- There is no data to support cytotoxic chemotherapy for the treatment of patients with very poor performance status (< 60% on the Karnofsky scale, or ECOG ≥ 3). However, patients with poor performance status and a known EGFR mutation may receive an oral EGFR tyrosine kinase inhibitor with a hope of clinical benefit without harm.

■ Duration of First-Line Chemotherapy

- The optimal duration of first-line chemotherapy remains a matter of debate.
- Some patients have progression of their cancer despite first-line chemotherapy and require immediate consideration of second-line chemotherapy.
- Randomized clinical trials studying duration of chemotherapy have failed to demonstrate a survival benefit for unlimited chemotherapy over a fixed number of cycles. However, the unlimited chemotherapy strategy clearly results in increased, cumulative chemotherapy-related toxicity.[41,42]
- Expert consensus is that all first-line chemotherapy will have diminishing returns over time, with cumulative toxicity. Therefore, few, if any, patients are eligible for chemotherapy beyond six cycles of initial combination therapy.[11]
- However, if the platinum is stopped, there is data to suggest that continuing the second drug may provide clinical

benefit (improved progression-free survival) without significant toxicity. This approach is called continuation maintenance therapy.

* Clinical trials validating this approach have been completed for gemcitabine and pemetrexed.[43-45]
* Taxanes and vinca alkaloids have not been tested in this regard because they are more likely to have intolerable cumulative toxicities such as peripheral neuropathy.
* The clinical trials that integrated bevacizumab or cetuximab into first-line chemotherapy also continued the monoclonal antibodies, as tolerated, until there was unequivocal evidence of disease progression, but whether continuation maintenance bevacizumab or cetuximab improves patient outcomes has not been established.[21,30]

■ Second-Line Chemotherapy

■ Docetaxel, pemetrexed (Alimta), and erlotinib are the only drugs with phase 3 randomized data demonstrating survival benefit in patients with recurrent or refractory NSCLC following first-line chemotherapy.
* One clinical trial randomized 373 patients with disease progression following platinum chemotherapy to receive either docetaxel (arm 1, $100\,mg/m^2$; arm 2, $75\,mg/m^2$) or vinorelbine or ifosfamide at standard doses (control arm 3).[46]
    ■ Patients who had received prior paclitaxel therapy were included in this trial, comprising about 40% of patients in each arm.
    ■ RRs to docetaxel were low—11% for arm 1 and 7% for arm 2—yet significantly higher than the RR with vinorelbine or ifosfamide, which was only 1%.
    ■ OS was not significantly different among the groups (approximately 6 months); however, 1-year survival rates favored the docetaxel-treated patients (32% vs. 10%, $P = 0.01$).
* A second trial randomized previously treated patients to receive either docetaxel or best supportive care.

- The objective RR to second-line docetaxel in this trial was 7%, similar to that observed in the previous trial.
- Treated patients experienced a significant improvement in median survival (7 vs. 5 months, P = 0.01).[47]
- Pemetrexed has been compared head-to-head with docetaxel in a large randomized trial of 571 patients with previously treated metastatic NSCLC.[48]
  - RR to each drug was 9% and OS was equivalent (median of approximately 8 months in both arms of the trial).
  - Pemetrexed caused significantly fewer side effects than docetaxel when both drugs were delivered at a high dose every 3 weeks.
- A randomized, placebo-controlled trial compared treatment with erlotinib with supportive care only in 731 patients with advanced NSCLC following failure of first- or second-line chemotherapy.[49]
  - Overall RR to erlotinib was 9%.
  - There was a statistically significant, and clinically relevant, difference in OS (6.7 vs. 4.7 months, P = 0.001).
- Other drugs, including gemcitabine and gefitinib, have documented phase 2 trial activity in previously treated patients, but phase 3 clinical trial data demonstrating a survival benefit over supportive care is lacking.
  - Gemcitabine was developed as a first-line drug, in combination with platinum, and has not been tested in phase 3 trials as a second-line drug.
  - A phase 3, placebo-controlled trial of gefitinib in previously treated patients with advanced NSCLC who were not selected for efficacy based on molecular or clinical characteristics failed to demonstrate a survival benefit of gefitinib over supportive care only.[50]
  - A similar trial that randomized previously treated patients between docetaxel and gefitinib attracted a more fit, less chemorefractory population of patients and was able to show equivalent efficacy between gefitinib and docetaxel in this population.[51]
- In summary, although second-line chemotherapy is reasonable in patients with good performance status, RR to

second-line chemotherapy is low (5–10%). The median survival of patients who make it to second-line therapy is 7 to 8 months.

- Similar to first-line chemotherapy, patients should not be administered second-line treatment until all critical sites of metastasis have been addressed (see Table 5.1).

■ Maintenance Chemotherapy

- Randomized trials have studied the effects of extended duration first-line chemotherapy in three basic ways:
  - Delivering a fixed number of additional cycles of two-drug chemotherapy
  - Continuing the nonplatinum drug beyond four cycles until disease progression, so-called "continuation maintenance"
  - Initiation of alternative chemotherapy immediately after four cycles and prior to disease progression, so-called "switch maintenance"
- Trials using docetaxel, pemetrexed (for those with non-squamous cell carcinoma), erlotinib, and gefitinib have shown increased PFS with switch maintenance therapy.[45,52–55]
  - In the study of pemetrexed and in one of two studies of erlotinib, overall survival (OS) was statistically significantly increased with switch maintenance therapy.[53,54]
  - In these trials, nearly one-third of patients in the placebo arm did not receive any post-study therapy despite the success of their first-line chemotherapy. As such, the OS benefit from switch maintenance chemotherapy seen in these studies may be related to inadequate treatment in the control arm rather than the added benefit of more treatment.
  - On the other hand, patients in the control arm may have become ineligible for additional therapy due to symptoms of disease progression. In other words, switch maintenance may be effective because it ensures exposure to second-line therapy before loss of patient fitness related to disease progression.

- The data on switch maintenance chemotherapy suggests that switching to a cytotoxic drug after four cycles of platinum-based chemotherapy appears to be more beneficial to patients with radiologic response.
  - Switch maintenance docetaxel is more beneficial in those who had prior responses (PFS: prior response hazard ratio [HR] 0.47, stable disease HR 0.81; OS: prior response HR 0.61, stable disease HR 1.02).[56]
  - Similarly, in the gemcitabine study, the benefit of maintenance gemcitabine appeared to be greater in those who had a response than those with stable disease (PFS: prior response HR 0.44 [95% CI, 0.31–0.63], stable disease HR 0.68 [95% CI, 0.48–0.97]).[45]
- In contrast, when patients are switched to erlotinib for maintenance therapy, this trend towards greater benefit in responders is less apparent.
  - Patients with radiologic response to first-line cytotoxic chemotherapy had no apparent benefit from switch maintenance erlotinib, while those with stable disease had more benefit than the overall study population (OS: responders HR 0.94 [95% CI, 0.74–1.20]; P = 0.618, stable disease HR 0.72 [95% CI, 0.59–0.89]; P = 0.0019).[54]
  - Sensitivity to initial cytotoxic therapy does not predict sensitivity to erlotinib, presumably due to its unique mechanism of action.[49]
- Any improvement in survival is tempered by increases in side effects.
  - The traditional approach remains to allow patients a break from cytotoxic chemotherapy after a fixed course of first-line therapy, with initiation of second-line chemotherapy at disease progression.
  - Ultimately, the decision of whether to use continuation maintenance, switch maintenance, or second-line chemotherapy must be made on an individual patient basis depending on a variety of factors, including:
    - Patient preferences
    - Patient fitness
    - Side effects from current chemotherapy
    - Pace or virulence of disease and disease burden

■ Molecular markers (such as EGFR mutation or ALK translocation), which may have been discovered during first-line cytotoxic chemotherapy and which may inform selection of subsequent drugs

■ Third-Line Chemotherapy and Beyond

■ Delivery of third-line chemotherapy, fourth-line chemotherapy, and beyond is limited by the cumulative side effects of chemotherapy and the increasing symptoms of progressive cancer, so that few patients maintain adequate fitness to tolerate salvage chemotherapy.

■ When the treating oncologist feels that the risks of harming the patient because of the side effects of chemotherapy are greater than the chance of clinical benefit, patients should be treated with supportive care only. A general algorithm for selecting chemotherapy for the treatment of patients with metastatic NSCLC is presented in Figure 5.1.

■ Surgery for Patients with Metastatic NSCLC

■ In general, patients with metastatic NSCLC—especially those with multiple synchronous metastases or metastases involving bone or liver—should never be treated with surgery with the intent to render the patient cancer-free.

■ Patients with stage IV NSCLC will likely develop other sites of metastasis in the time it takes to recover from a surgical procedure, and only chemotherapy has been shown to improve survival in these patients.

■ Surgery may be performed on a patient with incurable NSCLC with palliative intent (e.g., to drain a symptomatic effusion, repair a pathologic fracture of bone, or decompress the spinal cord in the event of a large vertebral metastasis when radiation therapy is not possible).

■ Some patients with a solitary metastasis to the brain or adrenal gland may be candidates for surgical removal of the metastasis (metastatectomy), with the intent to render the patient cancer-free.

   • There are retrospective case series of patients treated with surgical removal of a solitary brain metastasis or unilateral adrenal metastasis with good long-term survival.[57-59]

* Patients with a synchronous metastasis (i.e., the solitary adrenal or brain lesion is present at the same time the primary lesion is diagnosed) are less likely to benefit from metastatectomy than patients who develop a metastasis months, or even years, after the primary cancer has been treated—so-called metachronous metastasis.

* When faced with the decision of whether or not to treat a patient with a solitary brain or adrenal metastasis with curative intent, the patient's overall clinical course must be taken into account.

* A period of chemotherapy is often helpful to give additional metastases a chance to declare themselves prior to committing the patient to aggressive local therapy.

■ Radiation Therapy for Patients with Metastatic NSCLC

* Local symptoms from metastatic NSCLC can be relieved by a variety of doses and fractionations of XRT.

* For patients with severe chest symptoms (cough, hemoptysis, chest pain, lung collapse, SVC syndrome), radiation may be delivered to the chest at a low dose (i.e., < 60 Gy) with palliative intent.

* Randomized trials have tested whether to deliver palliative XRT to the chest early or late in the course of treatment, without clear differences in patient outcomes.[60]

* Radiation is also useful for the treatment of critical bone metastases or for the treatment of brain or spine metastases at doses of approximately 30 Gy delivered in 10 fractions.

* In appropriately selected patients, hypofractionated palliative radiotherapy (of 1 to 5 fractions instead of 10 or more) may provide symptomatic relief with acceptable toxicity in a more time-efficient manner.

■ References

1. Cullen MH, Billingham LJ, Woodroffe CM, et al. Mitomycin, ifosfamide, and cisplatin in unresectable non-small-cell lung cancer: effects on survival and quality of life. *J Clin Oncol.* 1999;17(10):3188–3194.

2. Thongprasert S, Sanguanmitra P, Juthapan W, et al. Relationship between quality of life and clinical outcomes in advanced non-small cell lung cancer: best supportive care (BSC) versus BSC plus chemotherapy. *Lung Cancer.* 1999;24(1): 17–24.

3. Non-small Cell Lung Cancer Collaborative Group. Chemotherapy in non-small cell lung cancer: a meta-analysis using updated data on individual patients from 52 randomised clinical trials. *BMJ.* 1995;311:899–909.

4. Group NM-AC. Chemotherapy in addition to supportive care improves survival in advanced non-small-cell lung cancer: a systematic review and meta-analysis of individual patient data from 16 randomized controlled trials. *J Clin Oncol.* 2008; 26:4617–4625.

5. Temel JS, Greer JA, Muzikansky, et al. Early palliative care for patients with metastatic non-small-cell lung cancer. *N Engl J Med.* 2010;363(8):733–742.

6. Hesketh PJ, Grunberg SM, Gralla RJ, et al. The oral neurokinin-1 antagonist aprepitant for the prevention of chemotherapy-induced nausea and vomiting: a multinational, randomized, double-blind, placebo-controlled trial in patients receiving high-dose cisplatin—the Aprepitant Protocol 052 Study Group. *J Clin Oncol.* 2003;21(22):4112–4119.

7. Kris MG, Hesketh PJ, Somerfield MR, et al.; American Society of Clinicagl Oncology. American Society of Clinical Oncology guideline for antiemetics in oncology: update 2006. *J Clin Oncol.* 2006;24(18):2932–2947.

8. Fossella F, Pereira JR, von Pawel J, et al. Randomized, multinational, phase III study of docetaxel plus platinum combinations versus vinorelbine plus cisplatin for advanced non-small-cell lung cancer: the TAX 326 study group. *J Clin Oncol.* 2003; 21(16):3016–3024.

9. Ardizzoni A, Boni L, Tiseo M, et al. Cisplatin versus carboplatin-based chemotherapy in the first-line treatment of advanced non-small cell lung cancer: results of an individual patient data meta-analysis. *JNCI.* 2007;99(11):847–857.

10. Schiller JH, Harrington D, Belani CP, et al. Comparison of four chemotherapy regimens for advanced non-small-cell lung cancer. *N Engl J Med.* 2002;346(2):92–98.

11. Azzoli CG, Baker S Jr, Temin S, et al.; American Society of Clinical Oncology. American Society of Clinical Oncology Clinical Practice Guideline update on chemotherapy for stage

IV non-small-cell lung cancer. *J Clin Oncol.* 2009;27(36):6251–6266.

12. Ettinger DS, Akerley W, Bepler G, et al. Non-small cell lung cancer. *J Natl Compr Canc Netw.* 2010 Jul;8(7):740–801.

13. Georgoulias V, Papadakis E, Alexopoulos A, et al. Platinum-based and non-platinum-based chemotherapy in advanced non-small-cell lung cancer: a randomised multicentre trial. *Lancet.* 2001;357(9267):1478–1484.

14. Kosmidis P, Mylonakis N, Nicolaides C, et al. Paclitaxel plus carboplatin versus gemcitabine plus paclitaxel in advanced non-small-cell lung cancer: a phase III randomized trial. *J Clin Oncol.* 2002;20(17):3578–3585.

15. Lilenbaum RC, Herndon JE 2nd, List MA, et al. Single-agent versus combination chemotherapy in advanced non-small-cell lung cancer: the cancer and leukemia group B (study 9730). *J Clin Oncol.* 2005;23(1):190–196.

16. Sederholm C, Hillerdal G, Lamberg K, et al. Phase III trial of gemcitabine plus carboplatin versus single-agent gemcitabine in the treatment of locally advanced or metastatic non-small-cell lung cancer: the Swedish Lung Cancer Study Group. *J Clin Oncol.* 200523(33):8380–8388.

17. Georgoulias V, Ardavanis A, Agelidou A, et al. Docetaxel versus docetaxel plus cisplatin as front-line treatment of patients with advanced non–small-cell lung cancer: a randomized, multicenter phase III trial. *J Clin Oncol.* 2004;22(13):2602–2609.

18. Scagliotti GV, Parikh P, von Pawel J, et al. Phase III study comparing cisplatin plus gemcitabine with cisplatin plus pemetrexed in chemotherapy-naive patients with advanced-stage non-small-cell lung cancer. *J Clin Oncol.* 2008;26(21):3543–3551.

19. Smith TJ, Khatcheressian J, Lyman GH, et al. 2006 update of recommendations for the use of white blood cell growth factors: an evidence-based clinical practice guideline. *J Clin Oncol.* 2006;24(19):3187–3205.

20. Rizzo JD, Brouwers M, Hurley P, et al.; American Society of Clinical Oncology; American Society of Hematology. American Society of Clinical Oncology/American Society of Hematology clinical practice guideline update on the use of epoetin and darbepoetin in adult patients with cancer. *J Clin Oncol.* 2010;28(33):4996–5010.

21. Sandler A, Gray R, Perry MC, et al. Paclitaxel-carboplatin alone or with bevacizumab for non-small-cell lung cancer. *N Engl J Med.* 2006;355(24):2542–2550.

22. Ramalingam SS, Dahlberg SE, Langer CJ, et al. Outcomes for elderly, advanced-stage non small-cell lung cancer patients treated with bevacizumab in combination with carboplatin and paclitaxel: analysis of Eastern Cooperative Oncology Group Trial 4599. *J Clin Oncol.* 2008;26(1):60–65.

23. Reck M, von Pawel J, Zatloukal P, et al. Phase III trial of cisplatin plus gemcitabine with either placebo or bevacizumab as first-line therapy for nonsquamous non-small-cell lung cancer: AVAiL. *J Clin Oncol.* 2009;27(8):1227–1234.
24. Maemondo M, Inoue A, Kobayashi K, et al. Gefitinib or chemotherapy for non-small-cell lung cancer with mutated EGFR. *N Engl J Med.* 2010;362(25):2380–2388.
25. Mok TS, Wu YL, Thongprasert S, et al. Gefitinib or carboplatin-paclitaxel in pulmonary adenocarcinoma. *N Engl J Med.* 2009; 361(10):947–957.
26. Mitsudomi T, Morita S, Yatabe Y, et al. Gefitinib versus cisplatin plus docetaxel in patients with non-small-cell lung cancer harbouring mutations of the epidermal growth factor receptor (WJTOG3405): an open label, randomised phase 3 trial. *Lancet Oncol.* 2010;11(2):121–128.
27. Lee JS, Park K, Kim SW, et al. A randomized phase III study of gefitinib versus standard chemotherapy (gemcitabine plus cisplatin) as a first-line treatment for never-smokers with advanced or metastatic adenocarcinoma of the lung. *J Thorac Oncol.* 2009;4(9):S283.
28. Zhou C, Wu YL, et al. Efficacy results from the randomized phase III OPTIMAL (CTONG 0802) study comparing first-line erlotinib versus carboplatin plus gemcitabine in Chinese advanced non-small cell lung cancer patients with EGFR activating mutations. *Annals of Oncology.* 2010;21(8):viii6.
29. Yang CH., Fukuoka M, et al. Final overall survival (OS) results from a phase III, randomized, open-label, first-line study of gefitinib v. carboplatin/paclitaxel in clinically selected patients with advanced non-small cell lung cancer in ASIA (IPASS). *Annals of Oncology.* 2010;21(8):viii1.
30. Pirker R, Pereira JR, Szczesna A, et al. Cetuximab plus chemotherapy in patients with advanced non-small-cell lung cancer (FLEX): an open-label randomised phase III trial. *Lancet.* 2009;373(9674):1525–1531.
31. O'Byrne K, Bondarenko JI, Barrios C, et al. (2009). Molecular and clinical predictors of outcome for cetuximab in non-small cell lung cancer (NSCLC): data from the FLEX study. *J Clin Oncol.* 2009;27(15s):8007.
32. Gatzemeier U, von Pawel J, Vynnychenko I, et al. First-cycle rash and survival in patients with advanced non-small-cell lung cancer receiving cetuximab in combination with first-line chemotherapy: a subgroup analysis of data from the FLEX phase 3 study. *Lancet Oncol.* 2011;12(1):30–37.
33. Pirker R, Paz-Ares L, et al. Epidermal growth factor receptor (EGFR) expression as a predictor of survival for first-line chemotherapy plus cetuximab in FLEX study patients with advanced non-small cell lung cancer (NSCLC). *J Thorac Oncol.* 2011;6(6s):S276.

34. Shaw AT, Yeap BY, Mino-Kenudson M, et al. Clinical features and outcome of patients with non-small-cell lung cancer who harbor EML4-ALK. *J Clin Oncol.* 2009;27(26):4247–4253.
35. Kwak EL, Bang YJ, Camidge DR, et al. Anaplastic lymphoma kinase inhibition in non-small-cell lung cancer. *N Engl J Med.* 2010;363(18):1693–1703.
36. Quoix EA, Oster J, Westeel V, et al. Weekly paclitaxel combined with monthly carboplatin versus single-agent therapy in patients age 70 to 89: IFCT-0501 randomized phase III study in advanced non-small cell lung cancer (NSCLC). *J Clin Oncol.* 2010;28(18s):5s.
37. Bunn PA Jr., Lilenbaum R. Chemotherapy for elderly patients with advanced non-small-cell lung cancer. *J Natl Cancer Inst.* 2003;95(5):341–343.
38. Ranson M, Davidson N, Nicolson M, et al. Randomized trial of paclitaxel plus supportive care versus supportive care for patients with advanced non-small-cell lung cancer. *J Natl Cancer Inst.* 2000;92(13):1074–1080.
39. Roszkowski K, Pluzanska A, Krzakowski M, et al. A multicenter, randomized, phase III study of docetaxel plus best supportive care versus best supportive care in chemotherapy-naive patients with metastatic or non-resectable localized non-small cell lung cancer (NSCLC). *Lung Cancer.* 2000;27(3):145–157.
40. Gridelli C. The ELVIS trial: a phase III study of single-agent vinorelbine as first-line treatment in elderly patients with advanced non-small cell lung cancer. Elderly Lung Cancer Vinorelbine Italian Study. *Oncologist.* 2001;6(Suppl 1):4–7.
41. Socinski MA, Schell MJ, Peterman A, et al. Phase III trial comparing a defined duration of therapy versus continuous therapy followed by second-line therapy in advanced-stage IIIB/IV non-small-cell lung cancer. *J Clin Oncol.* 2002;20(5):1335–1343.
42. Smith IE, O'Brien ME, Talbot DC, et al. Duration of chemotherapy in advanced non-small-cell lung cancer: a randomized trial of three versus six courses of mitomycin, vinblastine, and cisplatin. *J Clin Oncol.* 2001;19(5):1336–1343.
43. Brodowicz T, Krzakowski M, Zwitter M, et al. Cisplatin and gemcitabine first-line chemotherapy followed by maintenance gemcitabine or best supportive care in advanced non-small cell lung cancer: a phase III trial. *Lung Cancer.* 2006;52(2):155–163.
44. Paz-Ares L, de Marinis F, Dediu M, et al. PARAMOUNT: Phase III trial results of maintenance pemetrexed plus best supportive care (BSC) versus placebo plus BSC immediately following induction treatment with pemetrexed plus cisplatin for advanced non-squamous non-small cell lung cancer (NSCLC). *J Thorac Oncol.* 2011;6(6s):S275.
45. Perol M, Chouaid C, Milleron BJ, et al. Maintenance with either gemcitabine or erlotinib versus observation with pre-

defined second-line treatment after cisplatin-gemcitabine induction chemotherapy in advanced NSCLC: IFCT-GFPC 0502 phase III study. *J Clin Oncol.* 2010;28(15s):540s.

46. Fossella FV, DeVore R, Kerr RN, et al. Randomized phase III trial of docetaxel versus vinorelbine or ifosfamide in patients with advanced non-small-cell lung cancer previously treated with platinum-containing chemotherapy regimens. The TAX 320 Non-Small Cell Lung Cancer Study Group. *J Clin Oncol.* 2000;18(12):2354–2362.

47. Shepherd FA, Dancey J, Ramlau R, et al. Prospective randomized trial of docetaxel versus best supportive care in patients with non-small-cell lung cancer previously treated with platinum-based chemotherapy. *J Clin Oncol.* 2000;18(10):2095–2103.

48. Hanna N, Shepherd FA, Fossella FV, et al. Randomized phase III trial of pemetrexed versus docetaxel in patients with non-small-cell lung cancer previously treated with chemotherapy. *J Clin Oncol.* 2004;22(9):1589–1597.

49. Shepherd FA, Rodrigues Pereira J, Ciuleanu T, et al. Erlotinib in previously treated non-small-cell lung cancer. *N Engl J Med.* 2005;353(2):123–132.

50. Thatcher N, Chang A, Parikh P, et al. Gefitinib plus best supportive care in previously treated patients with refractory advanced non-small-cell lung cancer: results from a randomised, placebo-controlled, multicentre study (Iressa Survival Evaluation in Lung Cancer). *Lancet.* 2005;366(9496):1527–1537.

51. Kim ES, Hirsh V, Mok T, et al. Gefitinib versus docetaxel in previously treated non-small-cell lung cancer (INTEREST): a randomised phase III trial. *Lancet.* 2008;372(9652):1809–1818.

52. Fidias PM, Dakhil SR, Lyss AP, et al. Phase III study of immediate compared with delayed docetaxel after front-line therapy with gemcitabine plus carboplatin in advanced non-small-cell lung cancer. *J Clin Oncol.* 2009;27(4):591–598.

53. Ciuleanu T, Brodowicz T, Zielinski C, et al. Maintenance pemetrexed plus best supportive care versus placebo plus best supportive care for non-small-cell lung cancer: a randomised, double-blind, phase 3 study. *Lancet.* 2009;374(9699):1432–1440.

54. Cappuzzo F, Ciuleanu T, Stelmakh L, et al. Erlotinib as maintenance treatment in advanced non-small-cell lung cancer: a multicentre, randomised, placebo-controlled phase 3 study. *Lancet Oncol.* 2010;11(6):521–529.

55. Takeda K, Hida T, Sato T, et al. Randomized phase III trial of platinum-doublet chemotherapy followed by gefitinib compared with continued platinum-doublet chemotherapy in Japanese patients with advanced non-small-cell lung cancer: results of a west Japan thoracic oncology group trial (WJTOG0203). *J Clin Oncol.* 2010;28(5):753–760.

56. Fidias P, Novello S. Strategies for prolonged therapy in patients with advanced non-small-cell lung cancer. *J Clin Oncol.* 2010;28(34):5116–5123.
57. Billing PS, Miller DL, Allen MS, Deschamps C, Trastek VF, Pairolero PC. Surgical treatment of primary lung cancer with synchronous brain metastases. *J Thorac Cardiovasc Surg.* 2001; 122(3):548–553.
58. Bonnette P, Puyo P, Gabriel C, et al.; Groupe Thorax. Surgical management of non-small cell lung cancer with synchronous brain metastases. *Chest.* 2001;119(5):1469–1475.
59. Porte H, Siat J, Guibert B, et al. Resection of adrenal metastases from non-small cell lung cancer: a multicenter study. *Ann Thorac Surg.* 2001;71(3):981–985.
60. Falk SJ, Girling DJ, White RJ, et al. Immediate versus delayed palliative thoracic radiotherapy in patients with unresectable locally advanced non-small cell lung cancer and minimal thoracic symptoms: randomised controlled trial. *BMJ.* 2002; 325(7362):465.

CHAPTER 6

Treatment of Unresectable Stage III NSCLC

■ Radiation Therapy

■ Unresectable stage III NSCLC may be treated with high doses (≥ 60 Gy) of XRT with curative intent.

■ Patients with unresectable stage III NSCLC treated with single-modality XRT have a median survival of 9 to 10 months.[1]

■ Standard XRT with curative intent is delivered to outpatients, once per day, Monday through Friday, 1.8–2.0 Gy/day, to a total dose of at least 60 Gy (i.e., ≥ 30 treatments over approximately 6 weeks). Radiation oncologists can vary the way in which they deliver high-dose XRT.

  • In hyperfractionated XRT, the radiation is delivered more than once per day (typically two to three times/day) at a lower dose per fraction. The rationale behind hyperfractionation is that normal tissue is less likely to be damaged by a lower dose per fraction, while cancer cells are equally susceptible to both low and high doses per fraction.

  • In accelerated XRT, the radiation is delivered at a higher dose per week, either by increasing the dose per fraction or by treating the patient on weekends. The rationale behind acceleration is that cancer kill can be improved by decreasing the likelihood of cancer repopulation between radiation doses.

  • Continuous hyperfractionated accelerated radiation therapy (CHART) is a European XRT strategy that delivers radiation at 1.5 Gy per fraction, three times a day, to a total dose of 54 Gy over 12 consecutive days. Although this type of radiation may be slightly superior to standard XRT,[2] it is not commonly used in the United States because of the impracticality of delivering radiation three times a day and on weekends.

■ XRT can result in acute and delayed side effects, including radiation burns to the skin, esophagitis, acute or delayed radiation pneumonitis, and radiation fibrosis of the lung. Radiation pneumonitis may result in worsening of pulmonary symptoms (cough, shortness of breath) in the short term and/or chronic breathing difficulties in the long term.

■ Technologic advances for the delivery of XRT, including 3-D conformal treatment planning, intensity-modulated XRT (IMRT), image-guided, and respiratory-gated strategies, allow contemporary radiation oncologists to deliver a higher total dose of radiation to the cancer while limiting exposure to normal tissue.

■ Better technology and treatment planning has allowed for the delivery of higher doses of energy per fraction focused on the tumor and away from normal tissue.

• Hypofractionated radiation with a higher dose per fraction results in higher biological cancer kill, but is also more toxic to exposed normal tissue.

• Stereotactic body radiation therapy (SBRT) with hypofractionated treatment plans have been tested and proven to be effective, with good rates of local control, in patients with early-stage inoperable NSCLC.[3,4]

• Tumors that are close to the mediastinum and central airways may pose a safety threat, with unacceptable rates of pneumonia, inflammation, and bleeding observed in one phase 2 study.[5]

• The utility of hypofractionated radiation and/or SBRT in unresectable stage III NSCLC has not been established because it is more difficult to avoid normal tissues when irradiating mediastinal lymph nodes.

■ Chemotherapy Plus Radiation Therapy

■ Prospective, randomized trials have shown that patients with unresectable stage III NSCLC who are treated with chemotherapy plus radiation have improved OS compared with patients treated with radiation only.

- Patients with unresectable stage III NSCLC treated with two or more cycles of chemotherapy, followed by XRT, have a median survival of 13 to 14 months.[1]
- The chemotherapy may be delivered before radiation, during radiation, and/or after radiation.
  - In randomized trials, the best outcomes have been seen in patients who receive chemotherapy and radiation at the same time, so-called concurrent chemotherapy plus radiation.[6,7]
  - Patients with unresectable stage III NSCLC treated with two or more cycles of chemotherapy concurrent with XRT have a median survival of up to 17 months in randomized clinical trials.
  - The benefit of concurrent chemotherapy with radiation appears to be due almost entirely to improved local control of disease (i.e., that the chemotherapy can work as a radiation sensitizer while also treating micrometastatic disease outside the radiation field).[8]
  - The improved outcome of concurrent chemotherapy plus radiation results comes at a cost. Patients treated with concurrent chemotherapy plus radiation strategies have a much higher rate of acute side effects than those treated with sequential chemotherapy followed by radiation, including cytopenias with potential for life-threatening infection, as well as severe esophagitis that may require treatment delay and hospitalization for intravenous fluid support.
  - Patients must be carefully selected for concurrent chemotherapy plus radiation. Older patients, patients with low or borderline performance status, or those who present with profound weight loss are unlikely to complete concurrent therapy and are more likely to experience life-threatening toxicity.
- In order to more safely deliver concurrent chemotherapy plus radiation, some investigators have studied the use of lower doses of chemotherapy.
  - Recent randomized data suggest that low-dose, weekly chemotherapy, while adequate as a radiosensitizer, may be inadequate for the elimination of systemic metas-

tases, which adds to the survival benefit of concurrent chemotherapy plus radiation.[9,10]

* Consensus opinion is that, whenever possible, patients should be treated with a high-dose of systemic chemotherapy either before, during, or after XRT rather than dose-attenuated chemotherapy during XRT only.

■ Clinical trials are ongoing to investigate the utility of adding chemotherapy before (i.e., "induction" chemotherapy) and/or after (i.e., "consolidation" chemotherapy) the concurrent chemotherapy plus radiation.

■ Phase 3 data are currently lacking to establish a standard of care with regard to induction or consolidation chemotherapy.

* A randomized phase 2 trial comparing an induction plus concurrent strategy with a concurrent plus consolidation strategy demonstrated superiority of the concurrent plus consolidation approach.[11]

* A randomized phase 3 study showed that low-dose carboplatin plus paclitaxel followed by consolidation carboplatin plus paclitaxel was just as effective, but less toxic than cisplatin-containing regimens.[12]

* A randomized phase 3 trial failed to show the benefit of consolidation docetaxel following concurrent chemoradiation with cisplatin plus etoposide for unresectable stage III NSCLC.[13] This may have been due to the 7% rate of mortality associated with consolidation docetaxel in this study.

* A randomized phase 3 trial failed to show the benefit of consolidation gefitinib following concurrent chemoradiation with cisplatin plus etoposide and consolidation docetaxel.[14] As in the consolidation docetaxel study, results suggest the addition of gefitinib is more likely to be harmful than helpful.

* Current clinical trials are exploring the use of novel agents, such as the antifolate drug pemetrexed or the anti-EGFR monoclonal antibody cetuximab, when combined with radiation therapy.[15,16]

■ **Table 6.1** summarizes current standard regimens for the treatment of unresectable stage III NSCLC. Basic principles include:

* The best phase 3 data support high-dose cisplatin-based combination chemotherapy with etoposide or a vinca alkaloid concurrent with chest radiation and no evidence of benefit to consolidation chemotherapy thereafter. (*Continues on page 89.*)

Table 6.1   Selected Treatment Strategies to Combine Chemotherapy and XRT for Unresectable Stage III NSCLC

All radiation delivered in a single daily fraction on weekdays only.

Sequential strategies	Reference
Cisplatin 100 mg/m² IV on days 1, 29 Vinblastine 5 mg/m² IV weekly for 5 weeks, delivered on days 1, 8, 15, 22, 29 ≥ 60 Gy XRT, 1.8 Gy per fraction beginning day 50	1

Concurrent strategies	
Cisplatin 100 mg/m² IV on days 1, 29 Vinblastine 5 mg/m² IV weekly for 5 weeks, delivered on days 1, 8, 15, 22, 29 ≥ 60 Gy XRT, 1.8 Gy per fraction beginning day 1	2
Cisplatin 50 mg/m²/day IV on days 1, 8, 29, 36 Etoposide 50 mg/m²/day on days 1 through 5, 29 through 33 ≥ 60 Gy XRT, 1.8 Gy per fraction beginning day 1	3
Carboplatin AUC = 2 IV weekly for 7 weeks on days 1, 8, 15, 22, 29, 36, 43 Paclitaxel 45 mg/m² IV weekly for 7 weeks on days 1, 8, 15, 22, 29, 36, 43 ≥ 60 Gy XRT, 1.8 Gy per fraction beginning day 1 Carboplatin AUC = 6 + Paclitaxel 200 mg/m² IV × 2 cycles beginning after XRT	4,5

1. Dillman RO, Herndon J, Seagren SL, et al. Improved survival in stage III non-small-cell lung cancer: seven-year follow-up of cancer and leukemia group B (CALGB) 8433 trial. *J Natl Cancer Inst.* 1996;88:1210–5.
2. Curran WJ, Paulus R, Langer CJ, et al. Sequential vs. concurrent chemoradiation for stage III non-small cell lung cancer: randomized phase III trial RTOG 9410. *J Natl Cancer Inst.* 2011 Oct 5; 103(19):1452–60.

Table 6.1 continued

3. Kelly K, Chansky K, Gaspar LE, et al. Phase III trial of maintenance gefitinib or placebo after concurrent chemoradiotherapy and docetaxel consolidation in inoperable stage III non-small-cell lung cancer: SWOG S0023. *J Clin Oncol.* 2008;26:2450–6.

4. Belani CP, Choy H, Bonomi P, et al. Combined chemoradiotherapy regimens of paclitaxel and carboplatin for locally advanced non-small-cell lung cancer: a randomized phase II locally advanced multi-modality protocol. *J Clin Oncol.* 2005;23:5883–91.

5. Yamamoto N, Nakagawa K, Nishimura Y, et al. Phase III study comparing second- and third-generation regimens with concurrent thoracic radiotherapy in patients with unresectable stage III non-small-cell lung cancer: West Japan Thoracic Oncology Group WJTOG0105. *J Clin Oncol.* 2010;28:3739–45.

Table 6.2 summarizes outcomes for patients treated with various combinations of chemotherapy and radiation therapy in phase 3 trials. Additional chemotherapy after chemoradiation (so-called "consolidation chemotherapy") remains investigational, and has never been shown to improve survival compared to concurrent chemoradiation alone in a prospective randomized trial. However, some of the best survival outcomes have been observed in phase 3 trials in which all patients received some form of consolidation therapy.

Table 6.2 Outcome by Treatment for Unresectable Stage III NSCLC (Phase 3 Trial Data)

Treatment Modality	Median Survival	3-Year Survival
External beam radiation therapy alone (≥ 6000 rads)	10–11 months	<10%
Sequential chemotherapy using high-dose cisplatin-based combination, then radiation	13–15 months	10–20%
Concurrent radiation and chemotherapy using high-dose cisplatin-based combination	12–17 months	20–30%
Concurrent chemoradiation followed by consolidation therapy	23–35 months	30–40%

- Low-dose carboplatin-based chemotherapy has been delivered concurrent with chest radiation with intent to deliver full-dose chemotherapy after completion of radiation therapy.
- Concurrent chemotherapy plus radiation is more toxic than sequential chemotherapy followed by radiation. For patients with comorbid medical illness, poor performance status, clinically significant weight loss, or poor lung function, a sequential approach is preferred to avoid toxicity.

■ References

1. Dillman RO, Herndon J, Seagren SL, et al. Improved survival in stage III non-small-cell lung cancer: seven-year follow-up of cancer and leukemia group B (CALGB) 8433 trial. *J Natl Cancer Inst.* 1996;88(17):1210–1215.
2. Saunders M, Dische S, Barrett A, et al. Continuous, hyperfractionated, accelerated radiotherapy (CHART) versus conventional radiotherapy in non-small cell lung cancer: mature data from the randomised multicentre trial. CHART Steering committee. *Radiother Oncol.* 1999;52(2): 137–148.
3. Timmerman R, Paulus R, Galvin J, et al. Stereotactic body radiation therapy for inoperable early stage lung cancer. *JAMA.* 2010;303(11):1070–1076.
4. Timmerman RD. Surgery versus stereotactic body radiation therapy for early-stage lung cancer: who's down for the count? *J Clin Oncol.* 2010;28(6):907–909.
5. Timmerman R, McGarry R, Yiannoutsos C, et al. Excessive toxicity when treating central tumors in a phase II study of stereotactic body radiation therapy for medically inoperable early-stage lung cancer. *J Clin Oncol.* 2006;24(30):4833–4839.
6. Curran WJ Jr, Paulus R, Langer CJ, et al. Sequential vs. concurrent chemoradiation for stage III non-small cell lung cancer: randomized phase III trial RTOG 9410. *J Natl Cancer Inst.* 2011 Oct 5;103(19):1452–1460.
7. Furuse K, Fukuoka M, Kawahara M, et al. Phase III study of concurrent versus sequential thoracic radiotherapy in combination with mitomycin, vindesine, and cisplatin in unresectable stage III non-small-cell lung cancer. *J Clin Oncol.* 1999; 17(9):2692–2699.
8. Auperin A, Le Pechoux C, Rolland E, et al. Meta-analysis of concomitant versus sequential radiochemotherapy in locally advanced non-small-cell lung cancer. *J Clin Oncol.* 2010;28(13): 2181–2190.

9. Vokes EE. Optimal therapy for unresectable stage III non-small-cell lung cancer. *J Clin Oncol.* 2005;23(25):5853–5855.
10. Vokes EE, Herndon JE 2nd, Kelley MJ, et al. Induction chemotherapy followed by chemoradiotherapy compared with chemoradiotherapy alone for regionally advanced unresectable stage III non-small-cell lung cancer: Cancer and Leukemia Group B. *J Clin Oncol.* 2007;25(13):1698–1704.
11. Belani CP, Lee JS, Socinski MA, et al. Randomized phase III trial comparing cisplatin-etoposide to carboplatin-paclitaxel in advanced or metastatic non-small cell lung cancer. *Ann Oncol.* 2005;16(7):1069–1075.
12. Yamamoto N, Nakagawa K, Nishimura Y, et al. Phase III study comparing second- and third-generation regimens with concurrent thoracic radiotherapy in patients with unresectable stage III non-small-cell lung cancer: West Japan Thoracic Oncology Group WJTOG0105. *J Clin Oncol.* 2010;28(23):3739–3745.
13. Hanna N, Neubauer M, Yiannoutsos C, et al. Phase III study of cisplatin, etoposide, and concurrent chest radiation with or without consolidation docetaxel in patients with inoperable stage III non-small-cell lung cancer: the Hoosier Oncology Group and U.S. Oncology. *J Clin Oncol.* 2008;26(35):5755–5760.
14. Kelly K, Chansky K, Gaspar LE, et al. Phase III trial of maintenance gefitinib or placebo after concurrent chemoradiotherapy and docetaxel consolidation in inoperable stage III non-small-cell lung cancer: SWOG S0023. *J Clin Oncol.* 2008;26(15):2450–2456.
15. Vokes EE, Senan S, Treat JA, Iscoe NA. PROCLAIM: A phase III study of pemetrexed, cisplatin, and radiation therapy followed by consolidation pemetrexed versus etoposide, cisplatin, and radiation therapy followed by consolidation cytotoxic chemotherapy of choice in locally advanced stage III non-small-cell lung cancer of other than predominantly squamous cell histology. *Clin Lung Cancer.* 2009;10(3):193–198.
16. Govindan R, Bogart J, Stinchcombe T, et al. Randomized phase II study of pemetrexed, carboplatin, and thoracic radiation with or without cetuximab in patients with locally advanced unresectable non-small-cell lung cancer: Cancer and Leukemia Group B trial 30407. *J Clin Oncol.* 2011;29(23):3120–3125.

CHAPTER 7

Treatment of Resectable NSCLC (Stages I–IIIA)

■ Thoracic Surgery

- The cornerstone of therapy for resectable NSCLC (stages I-IIIA) is thoracotomy with complete surgical resection of disease and accompanying ipsilateral mediastinal lymph node dissection.

- Complete anatomic resection of the involved lobe(s) by lobectomy or pneumonectomy is superior to limited resection (wedge or segmental resection), with decreased risks of loco-regional recurrence, death by any cause, and death due to cancer.[1]

- Patients who are not candidates for lobectomy or pneumonectomy due to comorbid medical illness or limited lung capacity still benefit from limited resection of their disease.

- Video-assisted thoracoscopic surgery (VATS) allows surgeons to operate through smaller incisions in the chest wall.

  - Patients who undergo VATS have shorter recovery times and less postoperative pain than patients who undergo standard thoracotomy.

  - It is unclear whether thoracoscopic resection of NSCLC is equivalent to standard thoracotomy in terms of rates of cure.

- Patients with resectable NSCLC who are not candidates for even limited resection of their cancer due to comorbid illness (i.e., inoperable patients) may be treated with XRT delivered at a high dose ($\geq$ 60 Gy) with curative intent.

- Stereotactic body radiation therapy (SBRT) with hypofractionated treatment plans have been tested and proven to be effective in patients with inoperable early-stage NSCLC, with good rates of local control.[2,3]

- Tumors close to the mediastinum and central airways may pose a safety threat for SBRT, with unacceptable rates of pneumonia, inflammation, and bleeding observed in one phase 2 study.[4]
- Using needle-directed treatments, such as radiofrequency ablation (RFA) or cryoablation is another way to ablate inoperable small tumors.
  - These techniques have shown promise in safety and local control, but randomized studies comparing needle ablation versus external beam radiation versus limited resection are lacking.[5–7]
- For lack of data establishing the best technique for ablating of inoperable NSCLC, these alternative treatments (RFA, cryoablation, SBRT) must be prescribed on an individual patient basis and the decision shared by a multidisciplinary team.

■ Pancoast Tumor (NSCLC of the Superior Sulcus)

- NSCLC that invades the chest wall (T3) can still be completely resected by excising the involved area of chest wall and repairing the defect in the chest using prosthetic material.
- Similarly, tumors involving the diaphragm or structures within the mediastinum (T3) are resectable with appropriate surgical reconstruction.
- NSCLC of the superior sulcus is a special consideration for chest wall invasion because of the proximity of important nerves and blood vessels running from the neck across the top of the lungs.
- NSCLC of the superior sulcus are rare (< 5% of all lung cancers). They are often called Pancoast tumors, named after a prominent radiation oncologist who pioneered treatment of these difficult tumors in the 1920s and 1930s.
- These tumors arise in the lung apex and grow upward beneath the clavicle, often invading the brachial plexus and subclavian blood vessels. They also have a propensity to invade the chest wall.

- Due to involvement of critical structures, surgical resection of Pancoast tumors is often challenging or impossible.
  - Pancoast tumor is the one instance in the care of patients with NSCLC in which neoadjuvant therapy may be relied upon to improve resectability of the cancer.
  - Preoperative, concurrent chemotherapy plus radiation therapy followed by surgical resection for mediastinoscopy-negative (N0-1) NSCLC of the superior sulcus has been shown to provide the best long-term survival.[8]

■ Adjuvant Therapy

- Despite complete surgical resection, too many patients with resectable NSCLC develop recurrent cancer and eventually die of their disease.
- The higher the stage of disease, the more likely the patient will experience disease recurrence after surgery.
  - In nearly four out of five patients with recurrent NSCLC, the cancer will recur outside of the chest, in a distant metastatic site such as the brain, liver, bone, or adrenal gland.[9]
  - Such recurrence is due to invisible micrometastases present throughout the body at the time of surgery.
- Three randomized clinical trials of postoperative chemotherapy for patients with completely resected stage I–III NSCLC demonstrating absolute increases in 5-year survival rates of 4% to 15% over observation only have been published since 2003.
  - The International Adjuvant Lung Cancer Trial (IALT) randomized 1,867 patients with resected stage I–III NSCLC to three to four cycles of adjuvant cisplatin-based chemotherapy or to no chemotherapy.[10]
    - Chemotherapy consisted of cisplatin plus either etoposide, vinorelbine, vinblastine, or vindesine.
    - Both OS and disease-free survival (DFS) were significantly better in the adjuvant chemotherapy group compared with surgery alone.

- Overall 5-year survival rate was 45% in the chemotherapy arm versus 40% in the control arm, with a hazard ratio (HR) of 0.86 in favor of adjuvant chemotherapy (P = 0.03).
- Toxic side effects of chemotherapy during IALT included grade 4 neutropenia (17%), grade 4 emesis (3%), and less than a 1% rate of grade 4 neurotoxicity/ototoxicity and renal toxicity.
- Seven patients in the treatment arm (0.8%) died due to toxic side effects from chemotherapy.
- The National Cancer Institute of Canada JBR10 trial randomized 482 patients with completely resected stage IB–II NSCLC (excluding T3 N0) to receive four cycles of vinorelbine plus cisplatin chemotherapy or surgery alone.[11]
  - Grade 4 neutropenia was common, with febrile neutropenia in 7% of patients and two patients (0.8%) dying of side effects from chemotherapy.
  - Both recurrence-free survival and OS were significantly prolonged for chemotherapy-treated patients (OS, 94 months vs. 73 months; HR, 0.69; P = 0.011).
  - The 5-year survival rate for chemotherapy-treated patients was 69% compared with 54% for patients treated with surgery alone.
- A third study enrolled 840 patients with stage IB–IIIA NSCLC and randomly assigned them to observation or to cisplatin plus vinorelbine. Median survival was 66 months (95% CI, 47.9–88.5) in the chemotherapy group and 44 (35.7–52.3) months in the observation group. Adjusted risk for death was significantly reduced in patients assigned chemotherapy compared with controls (hazard ratio 0.80 [95% CI, 0.66–0.96]; P = 0.017).[12]
- The improvement in OS from adjuvant chemotherapy comes at the cost of hair loss, nausea, fatigue, and potential serious side effects, including permanent peripheral neuropathy, hearing loss, kidney damage, and lowering of blood counts, which increases the risk of life-threatening infection, with an approximate 1% risk of death due to infection or cardiovascular complication.

- Nevertheless, the high rate of recurrence for NSCLC following surgery justifies adjuvant chemotherapy for this disease, perhaps even more convincingly than for patients with resected colon cancer or breast cancer, diseases in which adjuvant chemotherapy is also a standard of care.
- None of the clinical trials listed here was able to detect the benefit of adjuvant chemotherapy exclusively in the subgroup of patients with stage IB disease. Using the old staging system, this includes any patient with a tumor > 3 cm in size with no lymph node metastases.
- Cancer and Leukemia Group B trial 9633 randomized 344 patients exclusively with lymph node negative stage IB (T2 N0 M0) NSCLC to receive paclitaxel plus carboplatin or no further therapy following complete resection.[13]
  - Paclitaxel plus carboplatin adjuvant chemotherapy was well tolerated, with no chemotherapy-related toxic deaths. Grades 3–4 neutropenia occurred in 36% of patients.
  - Despite an improvement in DFS and a trend to improvement in OS, this study did not demonstrate a statistically significant improvement in OS.
  - A subgroup of patients with tumors larger than 4 cm showed a statistically significant improvement in OS.
- A subgroup analysis from NCIC JBR-10 also demonstrated statistically survival benefit only in larger tumors > 4 cm.[14]
- A meta-analysis of all patients enrolled in randomized trials of adjuvant cisplatin since 1994 pooled more than 5000 patients and corroborated the benefit of adjuvant cisplatin in stage II–III NSCLC, but failed to show a statistically significant improvement in overall survival in patients with stage IB disease.[15]
- As a result of the lack of individual trials or meta-analyses showing a survival benefit of adjuvant chemotherapy in all patients with stage IB disease, expert consensus is that adjuvant chemotherapy should not be routinely recommended in stage IB.[16]
- Fourteen years after these adjuvant clinical trials were launched, the staging system for NSCLC was updated such that extremely large tumors (> 5 cm in size) are now

classified as T2b (stage II) even without evidence of lymph node metastases.[17]

■ Given this change in staging and subgroup analyses showing benefit in larger stage IB tumors, most would argue that adjuvant chemotherapy should be offered to all patients with stage II–III NSCLC regardless of lymph node status.

■ There is insufficient data to recommend adjuvant chemotherapy for patients with completely resected stage IA disease. In fact, the meta-analysis showed a trend toward harm from adjuvant cisplatin in this subgroup.

■ Furthermore, there is a lack of data to justify routine use of adjuvant cisplatin in elderly patients over the age of 80, in patients with poor performance status (ECOG $\geq$ 2, KPS $\leq$ 60%), or those who have serious comorbid illness.

■ Less toxic, more effective adjuvant therapies are sorely needed, especially for stage IA patients, for whom no adjuvant therapy currently exist.

   • Leading candidates for less toxic, more effective adjuvant therapies include vaccine therapies and molecularly targeted drugs.

   • A retrospective study of 167 patients with resected lung adenocarcinoma and EGFR mutation showed that the patients who received neoadjuvant or adjuvant EGFR tyrosine kinase inhibitor therapy had strong trends toward improvement in disease-free survival.[18]

   • The 2-year DFS was 89% for patients treated with adjuvant TKI compared with 72% in control group (HR = 0.53; 95% CI, 0.28–1.03; P = 0.06)

   • Randomized prospective trials of adjuvant EGFR tyrosine kinase inhibitors for resected NSCLC are planned.

■ Adjuvant Therapy and LCNEC

■ Certain large cell tumors express neuroendocrine tumor markers or have neuroendocrine morphologic features.

■ Large cell neuroendocrine tumors (LCNEC) are less responsive to chemotherapy and carry a worse prognosis compared with other types of NSCLC.[19]

■ Retrospective case series of patients with LCNEC treated with surgery show higher rates of recurrence and death even after successful surgery. These series suggest the need for more aggressive use of postoperative chemotherapy (adjuvant chemotherapy) for this histologic subtype.[20–22]

■ Neoadjuvant Chemotherapy for Resectable IIIA

■ Given the benefit of adjuvant chemotherapy delivered after complete surgical resection of stage IB–IIIA NSCLC, there has been increasing research interest in whether it is better to deliver the chemotherapy prior to surgery.

  • Patients are more physically fit before their surgery than afterward and are more likely to complete a prescribed course of chemotherapy.

  • The presence of the cancer in the chest gives the treating medical oncologist the opportunity to measure the patient's response to chemotherapy, allowing delivery of additional cycles of an effective regimen or early abandonment of an ineffective regimen.

■ Patients with clinical or pathologic evidence of stage IIIA (N2) disease should be referred for chemotherapy before surgery (neoadjuvant chemotherapy) as a standard of care.

■ There are numerous small, prospective randomized trials and retrospective case series showing improved survival versus surgery alone.[23–24]

  • A review of 136 patients with resectable stage IIIA (N2) NSCLC who received neoadjuvant chemotherapy with mitomycin plus vinblastine plus cisplatin prior to surgery reported a 77% major response rate, a 65% rate of complete surgical resection, and a 14% rate of pathologic complete response.[25]

  • Median survival for all patients was 19 months, with a 3-year survival rate of 41%, significantly better than historical controls treated with surgery alone (41% vs. 8%, $P = 0.001$).

■ Patients with a pathologic complete response to neoadjuvant chemotherapy are the ones most likely to be cured by surgery. This has led to clinical trials testing whether neoadjuvant radiation should be added to chemotherapy for patients with resectable stage IIIA (N2) disease.

- A randomized trial comparing definitive chemotherapy plus XRT (61 Gy), with chemotherapy plus XRT (45 Gy) followed by surgery for patients with resectable stage IIIA (N2) disease demonstrated a higher rate of early death in the surgery arm, likely due to the cumulative toxicity of combining all three treatment modalities.[26]
- Most of the treatment-related deaths occurred in patients undergoing pneumonectomy, such that existing data would suggest that preoperative chemoradiation followed by pneumonectomy is more likely to be harmful than helpful.

■ There was no difference in overall survival between the two approaches. A subgroup analysis showed that patients treated with chemoradiation and then lobectomy had better survival rates than matched patients treated with chemoradiation therapy alone. It is unclear whether this is because of the benefit of surgery or lack of treatment-related death in patients who underwent lobectomy.

■ Postoperative radiation therapy (PORT) to the bronchial stump and mediastinum decreases the risk of loco-regional recurrence.

- A meta-analysis of more than 2000 patients randomized to receive PORT or observation only for completely resected NSCLC demonstrated a survival decrease in the patients treated with PORT, especially for stage I–II patients, suggesting that PORT may be more harmful than helpful for some patients.[27]
- Results from retrospective data collected from a query of the Surveillance, Epidemiology, and End Results (SEER) database suggest benefit of PORT in stage IIIA disease. The large (n = 7,465) SEER retrospective study found superior survival rates associated with radiotherapy in N2 disease (HR = 0.855; 95% CI, 0.762 – 0.959).[28]
- A non-randomized subanalysis of the ANITA trial comparing 5-year overall survival in N2 patients who did or did not receive postoperative radiotherapy found higher survival rates in patients receiving radiotherapy in both the observation and chemotherapy arms (21% vs. 17% and 47% vs. 34%, respectively).[12,29]

- In summary, patients with N2 disease discovered at surgery have an exceedingly high rate of loco-regional recurrence despite complete surgical resection, and may garner survival benefit from PORT. Therefore, PORT is routinely prescribed for these patients.
- If PORT is prescribed for a patient who is a candidate for adjuvant chemotherapy, the chemotherapy should be delivered first. PORT should be withheld until all adjuvant chemotherapy is complete.
- For patients with a positive surgical margin (incomplete resection), PORT should be the priority to eliminate any residual cancer, followed by adjuvant chemotherapy as indicated.
- Whether patients with both a positive surgical margin and indication for adjuvant chemotherapy should receive concurrent postoperative chemoradiation remains a matter of debate. Only one study suggested benefit with this approach, and there is increased risk of dangerous toxic side effects such as esophagitis, pneumonitis, and neutropenic fever.[30]

■ In summary, the best way to treat patients with resectable stage III NSCLC remains an area of active research. Treatment options include:
  - Chemotherapy plus definitive XRT
  - Chemotherapy plus XRT followed by surgery
  - Chemotherapy followed by surgery with or without PORT, depending on the status of lymph nodes at resection
■ Neoadjuvant chemotherapy is a reasonable option for selected patients with early-stage NSCLC (stages IB–IIB).
■ Most of the clinical trials of neoadjuvant chemotherapy for earlier stages of disease (stage I–II) have had difficulties with patient accrual or early closure because of intervening publication of trials showing the benefit of adjuvant chemotherapy; this made it no longer ethical to randomize stage IB–II patients to surgery alone.
■ One negative, although instructive, clinical trial randomized patients with resectable stage IB–IIIA(N1) NSCLC to surgery alone, preoperative carboplatin plus paclitaxel, or postoperative carboplatin plus paclitaxel.[31]

- This study showed no difference in efficacy in the entire cohort; however, higher risk patients trended toward benefit only in the neoadjuvant arm.
- This study corroborated the fact that chemotherapy is better tolerated before surgery than after surgery—90% of the preoperative cohort completed therapy, while only 66% of the postoperative chemotherapy group completed chemotherapy.

■ A randomized trial of 355 patients with stage IB–IIIA NSCLC compared preoperative chemotherapy followed by surgery to surgery alone. The overall survival (OS) difference did not achieve statistical significance (P = 0.15), but median DFS was significantly better for the neoadjuvant chemotherapy arm (26.7 months vs. 12.9 months).[32]

■ Southwest Oncology Group (SWOG) trial 9900 evaluated neoadjuvant paclitaxel plus carboplatin in stages IB–IIIA versus surgery alone. The trial closed prematurely due to intervening discovery of the efficacy of adjuvant chemotherapy and was therefore not appropriately powered, though it did show a trend toward improved PFS and OS with neoadjuvant chemotherapy, and there was no difference in success of surgery between the two arms.[33]

■ A recent meta-analysis of all available randomized clinical trials evaluating preoperative chemotherapy in resectable NSCLC found improvement in overall survival in the neoadjuvant chemotherapy arm when compared with those in the surgery-alone arm with HR = 0.84; 95% CI, 0.77–0.92; P = 0.0001.[34] This level of benefit is identical to that seen in adjuvant chemotherapy trials and meta-analyses.

■ The preponderance of the evidence supports neoadjuvant chemotherapy for any patient whose clinical stage suggests they will merit postoperative chemotherapy (i.e., clinical stage II–III, and selected stage IB).

■ The major problem with neoadjuvant chemotherapy is inaccurate staging. There is a chance of false-positive lymph node metastases based on radiologic imaging (CT and PET scan) alone.

▪ The gold standard for detection of lymph node metastases is surgical resection. Because of the possibility of false-positive FDG-PET and CT scans for detection of lymph node metastases, it is the standard of care for patients with radiologic evidence of lymph node metastases to have tissue confirmation of N1–N2 disease by mediastinoscopy and/or endobronchial ultrasound (EBUS) and biopsy, and to rule out N3 (unresectable) disease.

▪ Given the possibility of false-negative mediastinoscopy and endobronchial biopsy, selected patients are treated for clinical node-positive NSCLC without pathologic confirmation of nodal status at the discretion of the treating physician.

▪ Given the complexity of clinical decision-making and variety of approaches to resectable stage I–III NSCLC, it is important that these patients be managed by a multidisciplinary team, including a qualified thoracic surgeon, medical oncologist, and radiation oncologist, with input also from radiology, pathology, and pulmonary medicine.

▪ A working algorithm for the selection of treatment strategy for patients with resectable NSCLC is presented in **Figure 7.1**.

Figure 7.1 Treatment of resectable NSCLC: multimodality therapy.

• A qualified thoracic surgeon should determine whether or not the cancer is **resectable**, and whether the patient is medically **operable**.

• Mediastinoscopy remains the gold standard for detection of positive lymph nodes due to an unacceptably high false-positive rate of CT scan + FDG-PET scan. EBUS is an alternative.

• A medical oncologist should determine whether or not the patient is a candidate for adjuvant or neoadjuvant chemotherapy, and which chemotherapy is best.

• This algorithm is based on clinical stage groupings from the seventh edition of the TNM classification of malignant tumors.[17] Black arrows indicate treatment strategies which are acceptable in routine practice. Gray arrows represent strategies which are acceptable in selected patients. All patients are encouraged to participate in clinical research protocols.

• For patients with resectable stage IIIA (N2) disease, there is debate whether they should receive neoadjuvant chemotherapy only, or neoadjuvant chemotherapy plus radiation, followed by surgery.

Figure 7.1 (continued)

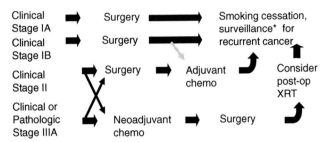

Selected neoadjuvant chemo options:
* Docetaxel + cisplatin × 3 cycles
* Gemcitabine + cisplatin × 3 cycles
* Pemetrexed + cisplatin × 3 cycles

Selected adjuvant chemotherapy options:
* Cisplatin (80–120 mg/m² every 3–4 weeks) + vinorelbine × 3–4 cycles
* Cisplatin 50 mg/m² days 1 and 8 + vinorelbine 25 mg/m² weekly every 4 weeks × 4 cycles
* Cisplatin 75 mg/m² every 3 weeks + novel agent docetaxel or gemcitabine or pemetrexed × 4 cycles
* For patients not eligible for cisplatin, a carboplatin doublet is acceptable × 4 cycles

*Surveillance after completion of all therapy should include history, physical examination, labs, and CT chest with IV contrast every 6 months for the first 2 years, and annually thereafter. After 2 years, annual non-contrast chest CT may be useful for the detection of second primary malignancies.

■ References

1. Ginsberg RJ, Rubinstein LV. Randomized trial of lobectomy versus limited resection for T1 N0 non-small cell lung cancer. Lung Cancer Study Group. *Ann Thorac Surg.* 1995;60(3):615–622; discussion 622–613.
2. Timmerman R, Paulus R, Galvin J, et al. Stereotactic body radiation therapy for inoperable early stage lung cancer. *JAMA.* 2010;303(11):1070–1076.
3. Timmerman RD. Surgery versus stereotactic body radiation therapy for early-stage lung cancer: who's down for the count? *J Clin Oncol.* 2010;28(6):907–909.
4. Timmerman R, McGarry R, Yiannoutsos C, et al. Excessive toxicity when treating central tumors in a phase II study of stereotactic body radiation therapy for medically inoper-

able early-stage lung cancer. *J Clin Oncol.* 2006;24(30): 4833–4839.

5. Lencioni R, Crocetti L, Cioni R, et al. Response to radiofrequency ablation of pulmonary tumours: a prospective, intention-to-treat, multicentre clinical trial (the RAPTURE study). *Lancet Oncol.* 2008;9(7):621–628.

6. Lanuti M, Sharma A, Digumarthy SR, et al. Radiofrequency ablation for treatment of medically inoperable stage I non-small cell lung cancer. *J Thorac Cardiovasc Surg.* 2009;137(1): 160–166.

7. Sharma A, Moore WH, Lanuti M, Shepard JA. How I do it: radiofrequency ablation and cryoablation of lung tumors. *J Thorac Imaging.* 2011;26(2):162–174.

8. Rusch VW, Giroux DJ, Kraut MJ, et al. Induction chemoradiation and surgical resection for superior sulcus non-small-cell lung carcinomas: long-term results of Southwest Oncology Group Trial 9416 (Intergroup Trial 0160). *J Clin Oncol.* 2007; 25(3):313–318.

9. Feld R, Rubinstein LV, Weisenberger TH. Sites of recurrence in resected stage I non-small-cell lung cancer: a guide for future studies. *J Clin Oncol.* 1984;2(12):1352–1358.

10. Arriagada R, Bergman B, Dunant A, et al. Cisplatin-based adjuvant chemotherapy in patients with completely resected non-small-cell lung cancer. *N Engl J Med.* 2004;350(4): 351–360.

11. Winton T, Livingston R, Johnson D, et al. Vinorelbine plus cisplatin vs. observation in resected non-small-cell lung cancer. *N Engl J Med.* 2005;352(25):2589–2597.

12. Douillard JY, Rosell R, De Lena M, et al. Adjuvant vinorelbine plus cisplatin versus observation in patients with completely resected stage IB–IIIA non-small-cell lung cancer (Adjuvant Navelbine International Trialist Association [ANITA]): a randomised controlled trial. *Lancet Oncol.* 2006;7(9):719–727.

13. Strauss GM, Herndon JE 2nd, Maddaus, MA, et al. Adjuvant paclitaxel plus carboplatin compared with observation in stage IB non-small-cell lung cancer: CALGB 9633 with the Cancer and Leukemia Group B, Radiation Therapy Oncology Group, and North Central Cancer Treatment Group Study Groups. *J Clin Oncol.* 2008;26(31):5043–5051.

14. Butts CA, Ding K, Seymour L, et al. Randomized phase III trial of vinorelbine plus cisplatin compared with observation in completely resected stage IB and II non-small-cell lung cancer: updated survival analysis of JBR-10. *J Clin Oncol.* 2010;28(1):29–34.

15. Pignon JP, Tribodet H, Scagliotti GV, et al. (2008). "Lung adjuvant cisplatin evaluation: a pooled analysis by the LACE Collaborative Group. *J Clin Oncol.* 2008;26(21):3552–3559.

16. Pisters KM, Evans WE, Azzoli CG, et al. Cancer Care Ontario and American Society of Clinical Oncology adjuvant chemotherapy and adjuvant radiation therapy for stages I-IIIA resectable non small-cell lung cancer guideline. *J Clin Oncol.* 2007; 25(34):5506–5518.
17. Goldstraw P, Crowley J, Chansky K, et al. The IASLC Lung Cancer Staging Project: proposals for the revision of the TNM stage groupings in the forthcoming (seventh) edition of the TNM Classification of malignant tumours. *J Thorac Oncol.* 2007;2(8):706–714.
18. Janjigian YY, Park BJ Zakowski MF, et al. Impact on disease-free survival of adjuvant erlotinib or gefitinib in patients with resected lung adenocarcinomas that harbor EGFR mutations. *J Thorac Oncol.* 2011;6(3):569–575.
19. Rossi G, Cavazza A, Marchioni A, et al. Role of chemotherapy and the receptor tyrosine kinases KIT, PDGFRalpha, PDG-FRbeta, and Met in large-cell neuroendocrine carcinoma of the lung. *J Clin Oncol.* 2005;23(34):8774–8785.
20. Saji H, Tsuboi M, Matsubayashi J, et al. Clinical response of large cell neuroendocrine carcinoma of the lung to perioperative adjuvant chemotherapy. *Anticancer Drugs.* 2010;21(1):89–93.
21. Iyoda A, Hiroshima K, Moriya Y, et al. Postoperative recurrence and the role of adjuvant chemotherapy in patients with pulmonary large-cell neuroendocrine carcinoma. *J Thorac Cardiovasc Surg.* 2009;138(2):446–453.
22. Iyoda A, Hiroshima K, Toyozaki T, et al. Adjuvant chemotherapy for large cell carcinoma with neuroendocrine features. *Cancer.* 2001;92(5):1108–1112.
23. Roth JA, Atkinson EN, Fossella F, et al. (1998). Long-term follow-up of patients enrolled in a randomized trial comparing perioperative chemotherapy and surgery with surgery alone in resectable stage IIIA non-small-cell lung cancer. *Lung Cancer.* 1998;21(1):1–6.
24. Rosell R, Gomez-Codina J, Camps C, et al. A randomized trial comparing preoperative chemotherapy plus surgery with surgery alone in patients with non-small cell lung cancer. *N Engl J Med.* 1994;330(3):153–158.
25. Martini N, Kris MG, Flehinger BJ, et al. Preoperative chemotherapy for stage IIIa (N2) lung cancer: the Sloan-Kettering experience with 136 patients. *Ann Thorac Surg.* 1993;55(6):1365–1373; discussion 1373–1364.
26. Albain KS, Swann RS, Rusch VW, et al. Radiotherapy plus chemotherapy with or without surgical resection for stage III non-small-cell lung cancer: a phase III randomised controlled trial. *Lancet.* 2009;374(9687):379–386.
27. PORT Meta-analysis Trialists Group. Postoperative radiotherapy in non-small-cell lung cancer: systematic review and

meta-analysis of individual patient data from nine randomised controlled trials. *Lancet.* 1998;352:257–263.

28. Lally BE, Zelterman D, Colasanto JM, et al. Postoperative radiotherapy for stage II or III non-small-cell lung cancer using the surveillance, epidemiology, and end results database. *J Clin Oncol.* 2006;24(19):2998–3006.

29. Douillard JY, Rosell R, De Lena M, et al. Impact of postoperative radiation therapy on survival in patients with complete resection and stage I, II, or IIIA non-small-cell lung cancer treated with adjuvant chemotherapy: the adjuvant Navelbine International Trialist Association (ANITA) Randomized Trial. *Int J Radiat Oncol Biol Phys.* 2008;72(3):695–701.

30. Lad T. The comparison of CAP chemotherapy and radiotherapy to radiotherapy alone for resected lung cancer with positive margin or involved highest sampled paratracheal node (stage IIIA). LCSG 791. *Chest.* 1994;106(6 Suppl):302S-306S.

31. Felip E, Rosell R, Maestre JA, et al. Preoperative chemotherapy plus surgery versus surgery plus adjuvant chemotherapy versus surgery alone in early-stage non-small-cell lung cancer. *J Clin Oncol.* 2010; 28(19):3138–3145.

32. Depierre A, Milleron B, Moro-Sibilot D, et al. Preoperative chemotherapy followed by surgery compared with primary surgery in resectable stage I (except T1N0), II, and IIIa non-small-cell lung cancer. *J Clin Oncol.* 2002;20(1):247–253.

33. Pisters KM, Vallieres E, Crowley JJ, et al. Surgery with or without preoperative paclitaxel and carboplatin in early-stage non-small-cell lung cancer: Southwest Oncology Group Trial S9900, an intergroup, randomized, phase III trial. *J Clin Oncol.* 2010;28(11):1843–1849.

34. Song WA, Zhou NK, Wang W, et al. Survival benefit of neoadjuvant chemotherapy in non-small cell lung cancer: an updated meta-analysis of 13 randomized control trials. *J Thorac Oncol.* 2010;5(4):510–516.

CHAPTER 8

Treatment of Small Cell Lung Cancer

■ Limited-Stage SCLC

■ Hematogenous metastases are so common in patients with small cell lung cancer (SCLC) that systemic chemotherapy is the cornerstone of treatment. In addition, the rapid rate of growth of these tumors typically requires haste in initiation of chemotherapy.

■ The staging system for SCLC (limited stage vs. extensive stage) is designed to identify patients who are candidates for thoracic radiation.

■ The role of surgery for limited-stage disease remains controversial.

• Surgery is typically reserved for patients with SCLC who have no evidence of N2–3 disease.

• Even if patients undergo complete resection of their SCLC, they should receive adjuvant chemotherapy.

• The overwhelming majority of patients diagnosed with SCLC have, at least, locally advanced disease not amenable to surgery.

■ Patients with limited-stage SCLC should be treated with radiation in addition to chemotherapy.

• A meta-analysis of more than 2000 patients treated with cyclophosphamide plus doxorubicin chemotherapy for limited-stage SCLC, with or without XRT, demonstrated a 5% increase in OS for the combined modality group.[1]

• Similar to strategies for the treatment of unresectable stage III NSCLC, chemotherapy can be delivered prior to, or simultaneous with, XRT.

■ In the 1990s, the combination of etoposide plus cisplatin (EP) chemotherapy gained favor as a regimen that was equally effective as the older, anthracycline-based regimens and was also better tolerated and safer to combine with XRT.

- Trials randomizing patients to concurrent EP plus XRT or sequential EP followed by XRT have demonstrated the superiority of the concurrent approach.[2,3]
- These trials also suggest that the earlier radiation is started in conjunction with chemotherapy, the better the outcome.

■ Patients with limited-stage SCLC treated with concurrent EP (four cycles) plus XRT to the primary tumor and associated lymph nodes (45 Gy, initiated on the same day as chemotherapy) have a median survival of 20 months, and nearly one in four patients are alive at 5 years.

- Hyperfractionated concurrent radiation, delivered in smaller fractions (1.5 Gy) twice a day, is superior to standard fractionation (1.8 Gy daily) with slightly superior survival in a head-to-head trial comparing these two approaches.[4]

■ Extensive-Stage SCLC

■ The majority of patients with SCLC (more than two-thirds) have evidence of distant hematogenous metastasis at diagnosis.

■ These patients should be treated with chemotherapy only, for four to six cycles, followed by repeat CT scan and MRI of the brain.

■ Randomized clinical trials have failed to demonstrate a survival benefit for high-dose or dose-intensive chemotherapy strategies, alternating drug regimens, or prolonged administration of chemotherapy beyond six cycles.

■ Similar to the treatment of stage IV NSCLC, first-line chemotherapy beyond six cycles yields diminishing returns and appears to achieve only increased cumulative toxicity. A list of selected chemotherapy regimens for the treatment of extensive-stage SCLC is presented in **Table 8.1**.

■ The RR of SCLC to first-line chemotherapy is excellent (> 80%). Although many urgent complications of NSCLC

Table 8.1   Selected Chemotherapy Regimens for the Treatment of SCLC

Regimen	Study
Etoposide 120 mg/m^2 IV over 60 min on days 1, 2, 3 Cisplatin 60 mg/m^2 IV over 60 min, once per cycle, on day 1 or 2 Repeat every 21 days	1
Etoposide 100–120 mg/m^2 IV over 60 min on days 1, 2, 3 Carboplatin AUC=5 IV over 30 min, once per cycle, on day 1 or 2 Repeat every 21 days	2
Irinotecan 60 mg/m^2 IV on days 1, 8, 15 Cisplatin 60 mg/m^2 IV on day 1 Repeat every 21 days	3
Cyclophosphamide 750–1,000 mg/m^2 IV over 30 min on day 1 Doxorubicin 45 mg/m2 IV push on day 1 Vincristine flat 2 mg IV push on day 1 Repeat every 21 days	4
Topotecan 1.25–1.50 mg/m^2/day for 4–5 days Repeat every 21 days	4

Shaded regimens constitute second-line (salvage) chemotherapy.

1. Turrisi AT 3rd, Kim K, Blum R, et al. Twice-daily compared with once-daily thoracic radiotherapy in limited small-cell lung cancer treated concurrently with cisplatin and etoposide. *N Engl J Med*. 1999;340: 265–271.
2. Skarlos DV, Samantas E, Kosmidis P, et al. Randomized comparison of etoposide-cisplatin vs. etoposide-carboplatin and irradiation in small-cell lung cancer. A Hellenic Co-operative Oncology Group study. *Ann Oncol*. 1994;5:601–607.
3. Noda K, Nishiwaki Y, Kawahara M, et al. Irinotecan plus cisplatin compared with etoposide plus cisplatin for extensive small-cell lung cancer. *N Engl J Med*. 2002;346:85–91.
4. von Pawel J, Schiller JH, Shepherd FA, et al. Topotecan versus cyclophosphamide, doxorubicin, and vincristine for the treatment of recurrent small-cell lung cancer. *J Clin Oncol*. 1999;17:658–667.

require immediate surgery or radiation therapy prior to initiation of chemotherapy, it is reasonable to treat oncologic emergencies from SCLC—such as threats to the spinal cord, painful bone metastases, or SVC syndrome—with immediate chemotherapy, in anticipation of brisk and reliable shrinkage of the tumor.

■ One exception to this treatment strategy is symptomatic brain metastases due to SCLC, which typically should be treated with immediate whole brain radiation therapy (WBXRT). Smaller or asymptomatic brain metastases can be treated with chemotherapy only, withholding brain radiation until the completion of first-line chemotherapy.

■ Despite an excellent rate of response to first-line chemotherapy, the majority of patients with extensive SCLC experience recurrence and eventually die of their disease. Median survival for patients with extensive-stage SCLC is 6 to 12 months, and 2% or fewer of patients are alive at 5 years.

■ For patients with disease recurrence at least 6 months after primary chemotherapy, retreatment with the same drugs may be considered.

■ For patients with disease that is refractory to first-line chemotherapy or that recurs 3 months or less after primary therapy, prognosis is very poor.

• Salvage chemotherapy is reasonable; however, RRs are only 20% to 25% for second-line chemotherapy.

• A phase 3 trial compared chemotherapy using topotecan (Hycamtin) with a traditional combination of cyclo-phosphamide plus doxorubicin plus vincristine (CAV) in 211 patients with SCLC who had relapsed at least 60 days after completion of first-line therapy.[5] Of note, approximately 30% of patients enrolled had received prior CAV.

• RR and OS were statistically similar between the two arms (24.3%, 25 weeks for the topotecan arm; 18.3%, 25 weeks for CAV). However, investigators were impressed with a higher rate of symptom improvement in the topotecan group compared with CAV, including significant improvements in dyspnea, anorexia, hoarseness, and fatigue.

* Grade 4 neutropenia was less frequent with topotecan, but anemia and thrombocytopenia were more common.

* Other drugs with phase 2 data against SCLC include paclitaxel (Taxol, Onxol), docetaxel, and irinotecan.

■ Prophylactic Cranial Irradiation

▓ Brain metastases are very common in patients with SCLC.

* More than 10% of patients have brain metastases at presentation.

* 50% to 60% of patients develop brain metastases at some time in the course of their disease.

▓ Prophylactic cranial irradiation (PCI), typically 30 Gy delivered to the whole brain in the absence of detectable brain metastases, reduces the risk of ever developing brain metastases and improves overall survival.

* A meta-analysis of survival data from seven clinical trials, including nearly 1000 patients randomized to receive PCI or observation only, demonstrated a decreased risk of death in the patients treated with PCI, corresponding to a 5% increase in survival at 3 years.[6]

* A prospective, randomized trial of PCI in 280 patients with extensive-stage SCLC showed that PCI conferred a significant reduction in the risk of symptomatic brain metastases (HR, 0.27; 95% CI, 0.16–0.44; $P < 0.001$) accompanied by improvement in overall survival from a median of 5.4 months up to 6.7 months after randomization. The 1-year survival rate was 27.1% (95% CI, 19.4–35.5) in the irradiation group and 13.3% (95% CI, 8.1–to 19.9) in the control group.[7,8]

* Irradiation had side effects but did not have a clinically significant effect on global health status.

* As such, PCI is routinely recommended to patients with both limited- and extensive-stage disease who achieve a complete response, or near complete response, following primary therapy.

- PCI may result in measurable neuropsychological deficits; patients with baseline neuropsychological problems prior to PCI are particularly susceptible.
- Although the benefit of PCI for patients who achieve a complete response or near complete response following primary therapy for SCLC is clear, the best way to integrate PCI into the overall treatment plan, as well as whether to offer PCI to patients over the age of 70 or those with underlying neurologic dysfunction, remains controversial.

■ References

1. Pignon JP, Arriagada R, Ihde DC, et al. A meta-analysis of thoracic radiotherapy for small-cell lung cancer. *N Engl J Med*. 1992;327(23):1618–1624.
2. Murray N, Coy P, Pater JL, et al. Importance of timing for thoracic irradiation in the combined modality treatment of limited-stage small-cell lung cancer. The National Cancer Institute of Canada Clinical Trials Group. *J Clin Oncol*. 1993; 11(2):336–344.
3. Takada M, Fukuoka M, Kawahara M, et al. Phase III study of concurrent versus sequential thoracic radiotherapy in combination with cisplatin and etoposide for limited-stage small-cell lung cancer: results of the Japan Clinical Oncology Group Study 9104. *J Clin Oncol*. 2002;20(14): 3054–3060.
4. Turrisi AT 3rd, Kim K, Blum R, et al. Twice-daily compared with once-daily thoracic radiotherapy in limited small-cell lung cancer treated concurrently with cisplatin and etoposide. *N Engl J Med*. 1999;340(4): 265–271.
5. von Pawel J, Schiller JH, Shepherd FA, et al. Topotecan versus cyclophosphamide, doxorubicin, and vincristine for the treatment of recurrent small-cell lung cancer. *J Clin Oncol*. 1999; 17(2):658–667.
6. Auperin A, Arriagada R, Pignon JP, et al. Prophylactic cranial irradiation for patients with small-cell lung cancer in complete remission. Prophylactic Cranial Irradiation Overview Collaborative Group. *N Engl J Med*. 1999;341(7):476–484.
7. Slotman BJ, Mauer ME, Bottomley A, et al. (2009). Prophylactic cranial irradiation in extensive disease small-cell lung cancer: short-term health-related quality of life and patient reported symptoms: results of an international Phase III randomized controlled trial by the EORTC Radiation

Oncology and Lung Cancer Groups. *J Clin Oncol.* 2009; 27(1):78–84.

8. Slotman B, Faivre-Finn C, Kramer G, et al. Prophylactic cranial irradiation in extensive small-cell lung cancer. *N Engl J Med.* 2007;357(7):664–672.

Treatment of Common Complications of Lung Cancer

■ Treatment of Brain Metastases

* Chemotherapy does not reliably treat brain metastases due to the presence of a blood-brain barrier that prevents most drugs from entering the central nervous system.

* Symptomatic or large brain metastases with surrounding edema require immediate therapy with corticosteroids to decrease brain edema and consultation with a neurosurgeon and radiation oncologist.

  * Although an immediate high dose of corticosteroids for severe, symptomatic brain edema may be warranted (as high as 100 mg of dexamethasone), most patients present with subacute symptoms and require less than 24 mg a day, in divided doses.

  * Prolonged, high-dose corticosteroid therapy (≥ 4 mg dexamethasone daily, or equivalent, for more than 1 week) should be accompanied by antacid medications to reduce the risk of gastritis or gastric bleeding.

  * A prophylactic antibiotic to prevent *Pneumocystis carinii* pneumonia (PCP) is also indicated in these patients, typically trimethoprim-sulfamethoxazole.

* Most patients with brain metastases are treated with WBXRT due to multifocal involvement in the brain.

* Patients with three or fewer brain metastases due to NSCLC (oligometastasis) may be candidates for surgical removal or for stereotactic radiosurgery (SRS).

* SRS involves precise focusing of external-beam radiation on a site of metastasis using three-dimensional treatment planning. SRS delivers a high dose of radiation to the tumor and minimizes radiation exposure to normal brain tissue.

- SRS may result in radionecrosis, in which the surrounding brain is unable to reabsorb the area of remaining necrotic tissue following ablation of the cancer.
  - Radionecrosis causes inflammation that may result in neurologic symptoms just as severe as, or even more severe than, the symptoms caused by the cancer and may require prolonged therapy with corticosteroids or surgical debridement.
  - For this reason, SRS is rarely, if ever, performed on brain metastases larger than 3 cm.
- Surgical removal of NSCLC brain metastases is typically reserved for:
  - Symptomatic solitary or oligolesions (i.e., 3 or fewer) easily accessible by the neurosurgeon
  - Dominant lesions resulting in critical mass effect that are too large to be treated effectively with radiation therapy
  - Critical metastases in the posterior fossa, where there is less space to tolerate radionecrosis
  - Critical or symptomatic lesions recurrent after radiation therapy
- Symptomatic brain metastases due to SCLC should typically be treated with WBXRT.
  - Solitary or oligometastases due to SCLC are uncommon, and most patients require whole brain treatment for micrometastases.
  - Small, asymptomatic brain metastases due to SCLC detected at baseline on the screening MRI can be treated with chemotherapy only, withholding brain radiation until the completion of first-line chemotherapy.
  - Even if patients achieve complete response in the brain to primary chemotherapy, PCI should be offered, even in the absence of measurable disease.

■ Treatment of Bone Metastases

- Bone metastases are critical if:
  - Bone pain is refractory to analgesics.
  - Vertebral metastases compress, or threaten to compress, the spinal cord, resulting in neurologic problems.

* Weight-bearing bones are threatened by pathologic fracture or pathologic fracture occurs.

■ Like critical brain metastases, spine metastases that compress the spinal cord can result in symptoms requiring immediate treatment with corticosteroids and consultation with a neurosurgeon and radiation oncologist.

■ Critical bone metastases are best treated with focal radiation therapy and/or orthopedic surgery.

■ There is data to suggest that the treatment of lung cancer patients with intravenous bisphosphonates, such as zoledronic acid (Zometa), reduces the risk of future skeletal-related events (SREs), including pathologic fracture and spinal cord compression, and the need for radiation therapy or surgery to bone.

* A randomized trial compared treatment with zoledronic acid with placebo in 773 patients with bone metastases due to solid tumors, the majority of whom had lung cancer.[1,2]

* The trial demonstrated that treatment with zoledronic acid was safe and significantly reduced the SRE rate at 21 months follow-up compared with placebo (36% vs. 46%, respectively; P = 0.023).

* The reduction in SRE rate was not accompanied by an improvement in OS. A subjective improvement in experience of bone pain, although implied by the results, was not reported.

■ Treatment of Pneumonia and Empyema

■ Patients with active pneumonia in a lobe of the lung where movement of air or mucus is trapped by proximal compression of the bronchial tree by tumor will not have their pneumonia cleared with antibiotics alone.

* Chemotherapy delivered to patients with so-called obstructive pneumonia may lead to lethal exacerbation of the pneumonia.

* If chemotherapy is indicated, these patients must be treated with radiation first to relieve the obstruction and release the infection prior to chemotherapy being considered.

- Patients with trapped infection in the pleural space (empyema) must undergo chest tube thoracostomy or surgical debridement to ensure the infection has been cleared prior to starting chemotherapy.

■ Treatment of Cough and Hemoptysis

- A chronic, nagging cough is common in patients with lung cancer.
  - Other common causes of cough—including infection, postnasal drip, gastroesophageal reflux disease, and ACE-inhibitor use—should be considered in a lung cancer patient before attributing the cough to cancer.
  - Cough due to cancer may be dry (nonproductive) or accompanied by sputum production.
    - A cough due to upper respiratory infection or pneumonia is typically accompanied by fever and purulent, green or dark-colored sputum.
    - Copious sputum production, so-called bronchorrhea, may occur in the setting of mucinous adenocarcinoma and/or pneumonic forms of lung cancer.
- Severe cough may result in chest ache, posttussive nausea and vomiting, shortness of breath, and insomnia.
- The best way to ameliorate cough or bronchorrhea due to lung cancer is to treat the underlying cancer with chemotherapy, radiation therapy, or surgery.
- There are a wide variety of medications available to treat cough symptoms.
  - Expectorants, such as guaifenesin, irritate the stomach and respiratory mucosa, thereby increasing respiratory tract secretions. This may loosen phlegm and thin bronchial secretions, making the cough more effective at clearing all secretions.
  - Anesthetic cough suppressants, such as benzonatate, work systemically (not topically) by anesthetizing stretch receptors in the lung that trigger cough. Benzonatate has limited utility against cough due to lung cancer.
  - The best antitussive medications are opioid analgesics, traditionally codeine or hydrocodone.

* Codeine may be delivered as 30–60 mg per dose, up to four times a day.
* If codeine is difficult to obtain, Tylenol #3 (contains 30 mg of codeine per tablet) may be used as a substitute.
* Opioid antitussives often cause side effects, including constipation and drowsiness. Hydrocodone may cause less drowsiness or constipation than codeine.
* Other opioids including morphine, methadone, and hydromorphone also have antitussive activity.
  * Guaifenesin preparations with codeine are also available, which allow coadministration of expectorants and cough suppressants.
  * Dextromethorphan is an analog of codeine that, like opiates, acts on the brain to suppress cough. Unlike codeine, this drug has little analgesic or addictive properties and is available over the counter in some cough medicine preparations, typically in combination with guaifenesin.
  * Inhaled bronchodilators, such as albuterol or ipratropium, may be useful to treat cough in patients with underlying obstructive lung disease or cough due to bronchospasm.
  * Rarely, corticosteroids may be used to reduce bronchial inflammation and improve the symptoms of cough.
* Hemoptysis, or coughing up blood, is perhaps the most distressing symptom that a patient with lung cancer may experience.
  * Mild hemoptysis may improve with a course of antibiotics to decrease endobronchial inflammation that may be exacerbated by bacterial colonization.
  * Copious hemoptysis must be addressed with radiation therapy or rigid bronchoscopy in an attempt to achieve endobronchial hemostasis.

■ Treatment of Venous Thromboembolic Events

* Venous thromboembolic (VTE) phenomena, including deep vein thrombosis (DVT) and pulmonary embolism (PE), are common in patients with lung cancer.

- If a lung cancer patient should develop peripheral edema that is asymmetric or acute, he or she should be referred for immediate Doppler ultrasound of the affected extremity to rule out DVT.
- Similarly, any acute onset of shortness of breath, chest pain, or hypoxia, in the absence of other obvious causes, should be worked up with a radiologic test, such as spiral CT scan with intravenous contrast or ventilation/perfusion (V/Q) scan, to rule out PE.
- A patient with active lung cancer who is diagnosed with DVT or PE should be treated with an appropriate dose of low-molecular-weight heparin (LMWH) delivered subcutaneously.
- There is data that supports treatment with LMWH indefinitely in patients with active cancer and VTE, without converting to warfarin anticoagulation.
  - A randomized trial compared the efficacy of subcutaneous injections of LMWH (dalteparin) and oral warfarin for the prevention of recurrent thrombosis (DVT or PE) in more than 670 patients with active cancer.[3]
  - The trial demonstrated that chronic use of dalteparin was more effective in reducing the risk of recurrent thromboembolism without increasing the risk of bleeding.
- Patients with active lung cancer and recurrent VTE despite therapeutic doses of warfarin should be treated with LMWH indefinitely.
- Inferior vena cava (IVC) filters to prevent PE in the setting of DVT have never been shown to improve survival in patients with lung cancer and VTE.
  - IVC filters may result in progression of clot distal to the filter.
  - IVC filters should be reserved for patients in the acute setting with active or high risk of bleeding, and in whom there is no other choice but to reverse anticoagulation.

■ Treatment of Malignant Effusions

* Approximately one of every four patients with metastatic NSCLC will develop malignant pleural effusion (MPE). Effusions are rarely seen in patients with SCLC.
* If the MPE is large or symptomatic, patients should undergo drainage of the effusion prior to starting chemotherapy.
* Large-volume thoracentesis provides temporary relief. However, MPE has the potential for rapid reaccumulation.
* Definitive treatment of MPE requires insertion of a chest tube via surgical thoracostomy, followed by fusing of the visceral and parietal pleura to eliminate the potential for fluid reaccumulation—so-called pleurodesis.
  * Pleurodesis can be achieved by injecting an irritant (typically talc or a sclerosing chemotherapy drug such as doxycycline) into the pleural space, either via the chest tube or during thoracoscopic surgery.
  * Pleurodesis results in severe inflammation, with accompanying pain, fever, and pneumonitis.
  * Patients undergoing chest tube thoracostomy and pleurodesis require prolonged hospitalization (typically 4 days or more), narcotic analgesia, supplemental oxygen, and close monitoring for at least 24 hours following pleurodesis.
* Patients who are not candidates for chemical pleurodesis may have an ambulatory pleural catheter inserted (Pleurx Catheter).
  * Pleural catheters allow frequent drainage of pleural fluid on an outpatient basis.
  * Prolonged apposition of the pleural surfaces, for several weeks in a row, may result in automatic pleurodesis (so-called pleural symphysis), without the need for talc or other sclerosing agents.
* Malignant pericardial effusion may result in cardiac tamponade.
  * Patients may present with hypotension or dyspnea in the absence of hypoxia, and physical examination reveals elevated jugular venous pressure with distended neck veins, distant heart sounds, and elevated pulsus

paradoxus (i.e., blood pressure decreases dramatically with inspiration, > 15 mm Hg).

* The diagnosis of cardiac tamponade is best confirmed with transthoracic 2-D echocardiography.

* Treatment of malignant pericardial effusion involves surgical drainage of the effusion, often with placement of a pericardial window to allow any recurrent fluid to escape into the pleural space.

* If a pericardial drain is required, the pericardial surface may be treated with a sclerosing agent to eliminate the potential for recurrence of fluid.

■ Treatment of Superior Vena Cava Syndrome

▓ Superior vena cava (SVC) syndrome due to NSCLC is best treated with EBXRT, which is the most reliable way to shrink NSCLC pressing on the SVC.

▓ Subacute SVC syndrome due to SCLC may be amenable to chemotherapy due to the high response rate of this disease to chemotherapy.

▓ SVC syndrome may result in upper extremity or jugular DVT, and prophylactic anticoagulation may be considered for patients with critical SVC syndrome.

▓ In situations in which radiation therapy is not possible, intraluminal stenting of the SVC may be performed by an interventional radiologist in order to palliate symptoms.[4]

■ Diagnosis and Treatment of Syndrome of Inappropriate Antidiuretic Hormone Release (SIADH)

▓ Patients may develop low serum sodium (Na^+), also called hyponatremia, for many reasons during the course of their disease. One possible cause is SIADH.

▓ Patients with SIADH demonstrate low serum osmolality (< 280 mOsm/kg), but high urine osmolality (> 300 mOsm/kg) in the absence of other potential causes of hyponatremia, including hypervolemia or hypovolemia. The hyponatremia may be asymptomatic or accompanied by nausea, anorexia, headache, restlessness, and/or confusion.

* SIADH due to lung cancer is best treated by treating the underlying cancer.
* Until the cancer is under control or ablated, patients should be instructed to avoid drinking water and to restrict their intake of all fluids to less than 1 L/day.
* Patients with severe hyponatremia accompanied by symptoms—such as severe confusion, convulsions, or coma—should undergo fluid restriction plus administration of hypertonic (3%) saline in an intensive care unit setting.
* Mild hyponatremia can be corrected with free water restriction only.
* If hyponatremia is chronic (48 hours), the rate of correction should not exceed 8–12 mmol/L/day to avoid cerebral demyelination syndrome.
* If restriction of free water and fluid fails to correct hyponatremia, the patient can be given demeclocycline, which damages renal tubular cells and induces nephrogenic diabetes insipidus, resulting in free water loss.
  * Demeclocycline doses range from 600–1,200 mg/day, by mouth, in divided doses.
  * Patients on chronic demeclocycline should be followed closely for photosensitivity, excessive drug-induced water loss and hypernatremia, and renal failure.

■ Diagnosis and Treatment of Hypercalcemia

* Most patients with lung cancer and high serum calcium (Ca^{++}), also called hypercalcemia, have active bone metastases.
* Some lung tumors release hormones that are analogues of parathyroid hormone, called parathyroid hormone-related peptides (PTHrPs). Lung cancers that produce PTHrP may result in hypercalcemia in the absence of bone metastases.
* Hypercalcemia is defined as a serum Ca^{++} level greater than 10.5 mg/dL, after correcting for hypoalbuminemia.
  * Because Ca^{++} binds to albumin, and only the unbound (free) Ca^{++} is biologically active, the serum Ca^{++} level must be adjusted for low serum albumin levels.

- To correct for an albumin level of less than 4 g/dL, add 0.8 mg/dL to the measured value of Ca^{++} for each 1.0 g/dL decrease in albumin.
- Hypercalcemia may result in lethargy; arthralgia; myalgias; abdominal pain; polyuria with volume contraction, which can result in prerenal azotemia or acute renal failure; and cardiac arrhythmia.
- The cornerstone of treatment for hypercalcemia is volume expansion with isotonic saline.
  - Once volume is restored, simultaneous administration of loop diuretics, such as furosemide, blocks Na^+ and Ca^{++} reabsorption in the kidney and may facilitate clearance of serum Ca^{++}.
  - Associated losses of potassium, chloride, and magnesium must be replaced if prolonged saline and loop diuretic therapy is required.
- Intravenous administration of bisphosphonates, including pamidronate (Aredia) and zoledronic acid (Zometa), inhibit osteoclastic bone resorption and are effective in the treatment of malignancy-related hypercalcemia.

■ Treatment of Pain

- Pain due to cancer may be mechanical, inflammatory, or neuropathic in nature and may be treatable with a variety of drugs, including narcotic and nonnarcotic analgesics, steroidal and nonsteroidal anti-inflammatory drugs, and neuroactive agents.
- Historically, cancer pain has been notoriously undertreated with narcotic analgesics for fear of causing narcotic dependency.[5]
  - Narcotic addiction should never be a consideration for the patient or physician in the setting of cancer pain.
  - Narcotic prescriptions should always be accompanied by instructions as well as prescriptions for drugs that prevent constipation.
    - Docusate is an anionic surfactant believed to stimulate intestinal secretion and increase the penetration of fluid into the stool by emulsifying feces, water,

and fat. A typical dose of docusate is three 100-mg capsules by mouth daily.

▩ A bowel stimulant derived from the senna plant acts directly on intestinal mucosa and may also act on intramural nerves and plexuses of the colon, increasing the rate of colonic motility. Senna may be taken as one to two tablets by mouth up to twice a day.

▩ Osmotic or cathartic laxatives—including lactulose, milk of magnesia, citrate of magnesia, and polyethylene glycol—may be necessary to treat severe or refractory cases of narcotic-induced constipation.

■ Treatment of Hoarse Voice

▩ Unilateral vocal cord paralysis can be remedied with surgical procedures that permanently fix the paralyzed cord in the center, allowing the opposite cord to move inward, oppose, and restore phonation.

▩ This can be accomplished by a procedure called medialization laryngoplasty, which is performed by a qualified head and neck surgeon.

▩ Intracordal injections of autologous fat or allogenic substances, such as Teflon, silicone, or collagen, can also be used to medialize the paralyzed vocal cord without the need for surgery.

■ Treatment of Dyspnea

▩ Due to the nature of lung cancer, patients with progressive disease often experience progressive shortness of breath (dyspnea) with exertion. Eventually, patients may even experience dyspnea at rest.

▩ The best way to treat dyspnea is to treat its underlying cause. Common, reversible causes of progressive dyspnea in lung cancer patients include:
  * Exacerbation of obstructive lung disease
  * Pneumonia
  * Pulmonary embolus
  * Anemia
  * Pneumonitis due to chemotherapy or radiation therapy

- Pleural effusion amenable to drainage
- Pericardial tamponade amenable to drainage
- Pulmonary edema related to congestive heart failure
- Lung parenchymal involvement by cancer amenable to chemotherapy
- Lung collapse due to cancer amenable to bronchoscopy or anticancer therapy

■ In the absence of reversible causes of dyspnea, symptoms may be controlled with supplemental oxygen and opioid analgesics.

■ Opioids, such as morphine sulfate, function as bronchodilators, anxiolytics, and analgesics and may result in both objective and subjective improvement in dyspnea.

■ Corticosteroids may be used to reduce inflammation around parenchymal lung cancer and may provide short-term relief of dyspnea.

- Patients requiring prolonged, high-dose steroids (> 20 mg prednisone or equivalent for a week or more) should also be treated with antacids for prophylaxis of gastritis and with antibiotics (trimethoprim-sulfamethoxazole) for prophylaxis of PCP.

■ Treatment of Anorexia

■ Loss of appetite, common in patients with lung cancer, is often a major factor in cancer-associated weight loss.

■ In the management of anorexia, it is important to first rule out or treat reversible causes of anorexia, including chemotherapy-induced nausea, constipation, or gastritis.

■ Effective anticancer therapy often results in resolution of anorexia.

■ Megestrol acetate (Megace) is a synthetic progestin that results in increased appetite and weight gain in patients with AIDS and cancer.

- The mechanism of action of megestrol is poorly understood, but it is believed to act centrally by altering brain neuropeptides.
- The typical dose of megestrol for lung cancer–induced anorexia is 800 mg daily, which requires the use of an oral suspension (20 mL of 40 mg/mL preparation).

- Megestrol has been associated with an increased risk of VTE (i.e., DVT) in some randomized trials in cancer patients.[6]
- Systemic corticosteroids also improve appetite.
  - The side effects of chronic corticosteroid use—including gastritis, immune suppression, elevations in blood sugar, and myopathy—preclude their routine use for the treatment of anorexia.
  - Patients with lung cancer often require systemic corticosteroids during chemotherapy or for the treatment of obstructive lung disease or pneumonitis, resulting in serendipitous improvement in appetite.

References

1. Rosen LS, Gordon D, Tchekmedyian S, et al. Zoledronic acid versus placebo in the treatment of skeletal metastases in patients with lung cancer and other solid tumors: a phase III, double-blind, randomized trial–the Zoledronic Acid Lung Cancer and Other Solid Tumors Study Group. *J Clin Oncol.* 2003;21(16):3150–3157.
2. Rosen LS, Gordon D Tchekmedyian NS, et al. Long-term efficacy and safety of zoledronic acid in the treatment of skeletal metastases in patients with nonsmall cell lung carcinoma and other solid tumors: a randomized, phase III, double-blind, placebo-controlled trial. *Cancer.* 2004;100(12):2613–2621.
3. Lee AY, Levine MN, Baker RI, et al. Low-molecular-weight heparin versus a coumarin for the prevention of recurrent venous thromboembolism in patients with cancer. *N Engl J Med.* 2003;349(2):146–153.
4. Urruticoechea A, Mesia R, Dominguez J, et al. Treatment of malignant superior vena cava syndrome by endovascular stent insertion. Experience on 52 patients with lung cancer. *Lung Cancer.* 2004;43(2):209–214.
5. Cancer pain relief and palliative care. Report of a WHO Expert Committee. *World Health Organ Tech Rep Ser* 1990; 804:1–75.
6. Loprinzi CL, Kugler JW, Sloan JA, et al. Randomized comparison of megestrol acetate versus dexamethasone versus fluoxymesterone for the treatment of cancer anorexia/cachexia. *J Clin Oncol.* 1999;17(10):3299–3306.

Malignant Pleural Mesothelioma (MPM)

■ Epidemiology

▪ Malignant pleural mesothelioma (MPM) is a rare cancer (< 3,000 cases per year in the United States) that originates in the pleura and is associated with exposure to asbestos.

* There may be a 20- to 30-year latency from asbestos exposure to onset of MPM. Incidence in the United States is estimated to have peaked in 2005, with more than 8 million Americans still at risk.

* Spouses of people who have worked with asbestos are also at risk for developing MPM because of second-hand exposure to asbestos, which clings to the clothing of asbestos workers.

* MPM not related to asbestos exposure may be related to SV40 viral infection. There is a high incidence of discovery of SV40 viral DNA in MPM specimens.

* Symptoms of MPM include chest pain, dyspnea, cough, and the effects of invasion of nearby structures, including Horner's syndrome and SVC syndrome.

▪ MPM grows and tracks along the pleural surface, resulting in circumferential pleural thickening around the affected lung, causing a pleural rind, illustrated in **Figure 10.1**.

▪ MPM is often associated with pleural effusion. Unlike NSCLC, MPM may still be surgically resectable despite an MPE.

■ Diagnosis and Staging of MPM

▪ The differential diagnoses of MPM include benign fibrous tumors of the pleura, pleural infection with reactive mesothelial hyperplasia, NSCLC, and secondary malignancies.

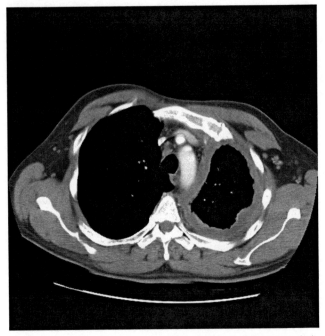

Figure 10.1 CT scan from a patient with malignant pleural mesothelioma (MPM) showing the characteristic pleural rind, and tracking along all pleural surfaces.

- MPM is most often diagnosed by way of thoracoscopic biopsy performed by a thoracic surgeon.
  - Needle biopsy of suspected MPM may result in insufficient tissue to make the diagnosis.
  - Direct needle biopsy of suspected MPM lesions may result in tracking of the tumor through the chest wall along the path of the needle.
- NSCLC may mimic MPM by growing in the pleural space, causing pleural thickening.
  - NSCLC and MPM can be distinguished by histopathologic characteristics including morphology and protein expression patterns on immunohistochemistry (IHC).
  - Unlike NSCLC, MPM tends to be negative for carcinoembryonic antigen (CEA) and positive for calretinin on IHC.

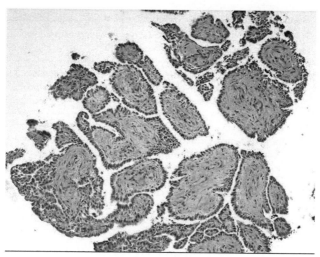

Figure 10.2 Malignant pleural mesothelioma.

- Electron microscopy may also help distinguish MPM from other types of cancer based on the distinctive shape and length of MPM cell microvilli. A photomicrograph of MPM under standard light microscopy is presented in **Figure 10.2**.
- Prognostic factors that predict poor outcome include higher stage, sarcomatous histology, poor performance status, severe pain, male sex, leukocytosis, thrombocytosis, anemia, and high LDH.

■ Treatment of MPM

- Treatment of MPM is guided by staging and whether or not the disease is resectable. The American Joint Committee on Cancer staging criteria for MPM are presented in **Table 10.1**.

■ Surgery

- Stage I–II MPM should be resected in patients for whom surgery is a viable option.

Table 10.1   Staging of Malignant Pleural Mesothelioma (MPM)

T1	Tumor involves ipsilateral parietal pleura, with or without involvement of the visceral pleura
T2	Tumor involves any of the ipsilateral pleural surfaces and is confluent with visceral pleural tumor, or invades diaphragmatic muscle or lung parenchyma
T3	Tumor involves any of the ipsilateral pleural surfaces and invades the endothoracic fascia, or mediastinal fat, or soft tissue of the chest wall; or exhibits nontransmural involvement of the pericardium
T4	Tumor involves any of the ipsilateral pleural surfaces, with diffuse or multifocal invasion of soft tissues of the chest wall, or any involvement of ribs, spine, pericardium, myocardium, brachial plexus, or invasion through the diaphragm to the peritoneum, or invasion into any mediastinal organs, or extension to the contralateral pleura, or pericardial effusion with positive cytology

Regional lymph nodes (N), distant metastasis (M)

Identical to NSCLC (see Table 4.1A, pp. 41–42)

Summary

T1–2 tumors are resectable.

T3 describes locally advanced but potentially resectable tumors.

T4 describes locally advanced, technically unresectable tumors.

Unlike with NSCLC, malignant pleural effusion from MPM is still considered resectable.

Stage groupings		Median survival (months)
I:	T1N0M0	30
II:	T2N0M0	19
III:	T3N0-2M0	10
	T1-2N1-2M0	10
IV:	T4 or N3 or M1	8

Adapted from Stahel RA, et al. Malignant pleural mesothelioma: ESMO clinical practice guidelines for diagnosis, treatment and follow-up. *Ann Oncol.* May 2010;21(Suppl 5):v126–8.

▪ Pleurectomy and decortication is a low-mortality, high-morbidity procedure in which the visceral and parietal pleura are literally stripped off the surface of the lung and chest wall.
  • Because the resection is piecemeal, there is a high rate of incomplete resection, and nearly every patient experiences local recurrence.
  • Frequent complications include supraventricular arrhythmias, pneumonia, and air leaks or fistulas.
▪ Extrapleural pneumonectomy (EPP) involves removal of the entire pleural surface, along with the ipsilateral lung, diaphragm, and pericardium.
  • EPP has a higher mortality rate than pleurectomy and decortication (5–10% overall), with equally high morbidity.
  • Although EPP provides for a more complete resection than subtotal pleurectomy, local recurrences are still common.
  • Recent retrospective studies have failed to demonstrate a survival benefit to patients with MPM who undergo EPP, and this type of radical surgery has fallen out of favor except in selected cases.[1,2]

▪ Radiation Therapy

▪ By removing the ipsilateral lung, EPP allows for delivery of adjuvant radiation to the chest with easier treatment planning and less observed toxicity because there are no vital organs remaining to be damaged by the XRT.
  • Adjuvant hemithoracic radiation can be delivered to a dose of 40–54 Gy, with a decrease in the risk of local recurrence.
  • Patients with MPM treated with EPP followed by PORT often have disease recurrence outside the chest, via direct extension into the abdomen or at distant metastatic sites. This has caused an increased interest in integrating systemic chemotherapy into the treatment strategies of patients with resectable MPM.

■ Chemotherapy

■ Patients with unresectable or metastatic MPM benefit from palliative chemotherapy.

■ A meta-analysis conducted in 2001 of more than 80 phase 2 efficacy studies concluded that cisplatin was the most active single agent against MPM, with an RR of about 20%.[3]

■ A randomized study of more than 450 patients with unresectable or inoperable MPM compared single-agent cisplatin with a combination of cisplatin plus the multitargeted antifolate, pemetrexed (Alimta).[4]

• The trial was amended after enrollment of the first 117 patients when investigators discovered that vitamin supplementation with oral folic acid and intramuscular (IM) vitamin B_{12} decreased the side effects of cisplatin plus pemetrexed, which include nausea, vomiting, neutropenia, and diarrhea. Severe stomatitis occurred in about 4% of patients.

• Patients in the pemetrexed arm lived longer (median survival 13 months vs. 10 months in the cisplatin-only arm) with an impressive phase 3 trial major radiologic response rate of over 40%, which translated into improvements in pain, dyspnea, and global quality of life.

• Patients with unresectable or metastatic MPM should be initiated on folic acid (1 mg oral tablet daily) and vitamin B_{12} (1 mg IM every 9 weeks) for at least 7 days prior to initiation of cisplatin plus pemetrexed. Pemetrexed is delivered at a dose of $500 \, \text{mg/m}^2$ IV over 10 minutes, followed 30 minutes later by cisplatin $75 \, \text{mg/m}^2$ IV over 2 hours, with the dose regimen repeated every 3 weeks.

• Patients who are not eligible for cisplatin may be treated with carboplatin + pemetrexed with similar efficacy and less toxicity.[5]

■ Other drugs with significant phase 2 trial activity against MPM include gemcitabine (Gemzar), which can also be combined with cisplatin or carboplatin for treatment of MPM,[6-8] as well as single-agent vinorelbine (Navelbine).[9,10]

▪ The combination of pemetrexed plus cisplatin chemotherapy has been studied as neoadjuvant therapy for patients with resectable MPM to decrease risk of distant metastatic recurrence, followed by EPP plus PORT.[11] Median survival was 17 months (95% CI, 14 to 23 months) with the best outcomes seen in patients who were able to complete all three treatment modalities.

■ References

1. Flores RM. Surgical options in malignant pleural mesothelioma: extrapleural pneumonectomy or pleurectomy/decortication. *Semin Thorac Cardiovasc Surg.* 2009;21(2):149–153.
2. Flores RM, Pass HI, Seshan VE, et al. Extrapleural pneumonectomy versus pleurectomy/decortication in the surgical management of malignant pleural mesothelioma: results in 663 patients. *J Thorac Cardiovasc Surg.* 2008;135(3):620–626, 626 e621–623.
3. Berghmans T, Paesmans M, Lalami Y, et al. Activity of chemotherapy and immunotherapy on malignant mesothelioma: a systematic review of the literature with meta-analysis. *Lung Cancer.* 2002;38(2):111–121.
4. Vogelzang NJ, Rusthoven JJ, Symanowski J, et al. Phase III study of pemetrexed in combination with cisplatin versus cisplatin alone in patients with malignant pleural mesothelioma. *J Clin Oncol.* 2003;21(14):2636–2644.
5. Santoro A, O'Brien ME, Stahel RA, et al. Pemetrexed plus cisplatin or pemetrexed plus carboplatin for chemonaive patients with malignant pleural mesothelioma: results of the International Expanded Access Program. *J Thorac Oncol.* 2008;3(7):756–763.
6. Favaretto AG, Aversa SM, Paccagnella A, et al. Gemcitabine combined with carboplatin in patients with malignant pleural mesothelioma: a multicentric phase II study. *Cancer.* 2003;97(11):2791–2797.
7. Nowak AK, Byrne MJ, Williamson R, et al. A multicentre phase II study of cisplatin and gemcitabine for malignant mesothelioma. *Br J Cancer.* 2002;87(5):491–496.
8. Byrne MJ, Davidson JA, Musk AW, et al. Cisplatin and gemcitabine treatment for malignant mesothelioma: a phase II study. *J Clin Oncol.* 1999;17(1):25–30.
9. Stebbing J, Powles T, McPherson, et al. The efficacy and safety of weekly vinorelbine in relapsed malignant pleural mesothelioma. *Lung Cancer.* 2009;63(1):94–97.
10. Steele JP, Shamash J, Evans MT, et al. Phase II study of vinorelbine in patients with malignant pleural mesothelioma. *J Clin Oncol.* 2000;18(23):3912–3917.

11. Krug LM, Pass HI, Rusch VW, et al. Multicenter phase II trial of neoadjuvant pemetrexed plus cisplatin followed by extrapleural pneumonectomy and radiation for malignant pleural mesothelioma. *J Clin Oncol.* 2009;27(18): 3007–3013.

CHAPTER 11

Malignant Thymoma

■ Diagnosis and Staging of Malignant Thymoma

* The thymus is a gland located in the anterior mediastinum and made up of epithelial, immune, and neuroendocrine cells; it is involved in the development of the immune system.

* Malignant thymoma is a rare tumor originating in the thymus gland.

* It usually presents with symptoms of pleuritic chest pain, chest ache, cough, and/or shortness of breath, with imaging studies revealing a mass in the anterior mediastinum.

  * Anterior mediastinal masses are usually malignant and limited differential diagnosis includes thymoma, lymphoma, inferior extension of a thyroid tumor, and germ cell tumor.

  * Thymomas are the most common of these, representing at least 30% of all anterior mediastinal masses.

  * Fine-needle aspiration may not be sufficient to differentiate the above tumor types; therefore, surgical biopsy or core needle biopsy may be necessary.

  * There is some evidence that disruption of the thymic capsule increases the risk of metastasis of malignant thymoma, such that some surgeons prefer complete surgical resection of an anterior mediastinal mass rather than core needle biopsy if there is a strong clinical suspicion of thymoma.

* Thymomas originate from thymic epithelial cells and not from the lymphoid cells populating the organ during their maturation.

  * They are composed of cells that have a histologically bland appearance and resemble normal thymic epithelial cells.

  * Thymomas can be classified by cortical, medullary, or mixed type, depending on the degree of similarity of

137

the cells with normal cortical or medullary thymic counterparts. Thymomas have variable amounts of lymphoid tissue associated with them.

▪ The behavior of a malignant thymoma is as important as histopathology to overall prognosis.

• A thymoma with a bland appearance that is actively invading the thymic capsule or adjacent structures or actively metastasizing throughout the chest may have a worse prognosis than a thymoma that appears histologically more aggressive but is contained within the thymic capsule.

• Thymic carcinomas are a subcategory of malignant thymoma that are composed of cells with a poorly differentiated, nonthymic appearance under the microscope.

• Thymic carcinomas share an invasiveness and a metastatic potential similar to NSCLC.

• Malignant thymomas are highly responsive to chemotherapy, while thymic carcinomas are notoriously chemoresistant.

▪ Nearly two-thirds of patients with thymoma have an associated autoimmune disorder, with possibilities including myasthenia gravis, Eaton-Lambert syndrome, polymyositis, pure red cell aplasia, hypogammaglobulinemia, pernicious anemia, panhypopituitarism, Hashimoto's thyroiditis, Graves' disease, Addison's disease, systemic lupus erythematosus, Sjögren's syndrome, rheumatoid arthritis, scleroderma, and nephrotic syndrome.[1]

▪ Myasthenia gravis is the most common autoimmune disorder, occurring in one out of every three patients with thymoma.

• Patients with myasthenia gravis should be carefully screened prior to surgery because of the possibility of perioperative respiratory complications.

• Treatment of the thymoma may improve the associated autoimmune syndrome, but not always.

▪ Thymomas are staged according to a system proposed by Masaoka more than 30 years ago.[2]

• Thymomas without capsular invasion are stage I (5-year survival rate, 93%).

* Invasion through the capsule into surrounding fatty tissue is stage II (5-year survival rate, 86%).
* Direct invasion into a surrounding organ is stage III (5-year survival rate, 70%).
* Pleural or pericardial dissemination, or lymphogenous or hematogenous metastasis, constitutes stage IV (5-year survival rate, 50%).

■ Treatment of Malignant Thymoma

■ Surgery is the mainstay of treatment for stages I–III malignant thymoma.
  * The initial resection should be done through a median sternotomy, with as complete a thymectomy as possible.
  * Given that the growth pattern of malignant thymoma may be indolent, recurrent thymoma may be amenable to repeat surgical resections over time, including resection of metastatic deposits within the chest, with good long-term survival.
■ No adjuvant therapy is required for stage I disease following a complete surgical resection.
■ Adjuvant radiation therapy is recommended for patients with stage III disease.
■ Adjuvant radiation is controversial for patients with stage II disease, especially those with only microscopic capsular invasion.
■ Some patients with locally advanced (stage III–IV) disease may be treated with adjuvant chemotherapy and radiation therapy following surgery.
■ Neoadjuvant chemotherapy and radiation may improve resectability of locally advanced thymoma.[3,4]
■ Patients with stage IV disease not amenable to complete surgical resection are treated with chemotherapy with palliative intent.
  * There are no prospective randomized trials comparing different chemotherapeutic agents.
  * Both single-drug and combination regimens have been used, with RRs as high as 90% in some phase II trials.[1]

- Cisplatin, the most commonly used drug, can be combined with etoposide (EP) or with cyclophosphamide plus doxorubicin (CAP) with good efficacy.
- Thymomas have been found incidentally to express receptors for somatostatin (SST) and to light up on SST-receptor scintigraphy with radiolabeled octreotide (octreoscans).
- There are case reports and phase 2 trial efficacy data that suggest therapeutic benefit in treating octreoscan-positive metastatic thymomas with subcutaneous injections of octreotide, with or without corticosteroids.[5,6]
- Side effects of octreotide include abdominal cramps and discomfort, constipation, diarrhea, flatulence, and nausea.

■ References

1. Johnson SB, Eng TY, Giaccone G, Thomas CR Jr. Thymoma: update for the new millennium. *Oncologist.* 2001;6(3):239–246.
2. Masaoka A, Monden Y, Nakahara K, Tanioka T. Follow-up study of thymomas with special reference to their clinical stages. *Cancer,* 1981;48(11):2485–2492.
3. Venuta F, Rendina EA, Longo F, et al. Long-term outcome after multimodality treatment for stage III thymic tumors. *Ann Thorac Surg.* 2003;76(6):1866–1872; discussion 1872.
4. Shin DM, Walsh, Komaki R, et al. A multidisciplinary approach to therapy for unresectable malignant thymoma. *Ann Intern Med.* 1998;129(2):100–104.
5. Loehrer PJ, Sr, Wang W, Johnson DH, et al. Eastern Cooperative Oncology Group Phase II Trail. Octreotide alone or with prednisone in patients with advanced thymoma and thymic carcinoma: an Eastern Cooperative Oncology Group Phase II Trial. *J Clin Oncol.* 2004;22(2):293–299.
6. Palmieri G, Lastoria S, Colao A, et al. Successful treatment of a patient with a thymoma and pure red-cell aplasia with octreotide and prednisone. *N Engl J Med.* 1997;336(4):263–265.

CHAPTER 12

What the Future Holds

■ 2012 Update

- Screening for lung cancer in heavy smokers using low-dose CT scan will result in a rise in the incidence (discovery) of early-stage lung cancer. This will decrease lung cancer mortality and increase the importance of diagnostic and therapeutic techniques for early-stage lung cancer.

- It remains to be seen which discipline will take the lead in caring for all these new patients, who traditionally have been managed by thoracic surgeons but in the future may be referred more frequently to radiation oncologists or interventional radiologists for non invasive or minimally invasive therapeutics.

- The rising incidence of early-stage lung cancer will increase the importance for development of prognostic and predictive molecular markers and adjuvant therapies, including more effective and less toxic drugs, as well as vaccine therapies.

- As our knowledge increases regarding the molecular mechanisms that drive lung cancer, we are becoming more dependent on molecular classification of the disease to select treatment strategies.

- In addition to EGFR (HER1) and ALK, druggable oncogene targets in lung cancer with ongoing phase 1–3 clinical trials include VEGFR, IGF1R, MET, HER2, HER3, PI3K, AKT, MEK, and mTOR.

- With the discovery of EGFR-activating mutations in 10% of all patients with NSCLC and EGFR tyrosine kinase inhibitors that effectively target these driver mutations, we have established this subtype of NSCLC as an independent disease, worthy of unique and independent treatment pathways.

- Patients with NSCLC and EGFR-activating mutation have a better prognosis regardless of therapy, so identification of these patients is vital to interpretation of clinical trial results.
- These patients develop acquired resistance to EGFR tyrosine kinase inhibitors, with specific molecular determinants of resistance, such as EGFR T790M or MET amplification, which may be treatable with alternative targeted drugs.
- Clinical trials are now focusing on the many patients per year (20,000+ per year in the United States) who develop acquired resistance to erlotinib.
- This pathway of disease with a druggable oncogene with established pathways of acquired molecular resistance is akin to the treatment of chronic myelogenous leukemia (CML) with drugs targeting abl kinase, except there are 10 times as many patients with EGFR mutant lung cancer than there are with CML.
■ Discovery of the 3–5% of patients with NSCLC driven by EML4-ALK translocation and treatable with ALK inhibitors like crizotinib is the most recently discovered unique subtype of NSCLC, which should be treated with different drugs than used with other patients with NSCLC.
  - The FDA recently approved crizotinib (Xalkori) for patients with stage IV NSCLC and ALK translocation.
  - Clinical trials testing first-line use of crizotinib and new drugs for patients with acquired resistance to crizotinib are ongoing.
■ Discovery that even cytotoxic chemotherapy has differential efficacy in subgroups of NSCLC has led to increased importance of better classifying NSCLC as adenocarcinoma, squamous carcinoma, and LCNEC using closer scrutiny of morphologic and immunohistochemical characteristics.
■ The term *non-small cell lung cancer* will fall out of favor as an obsolete classification based on exclusion. Similarly, the term *nonsquamous* will fall out of favor as an obsolete classification of exclusion once the molecular determinants

of the differentical efficacy of pemetrexed in this subgroup are discovered.

- Molecular predictors of benefit from antiangiogenesis drugs will be discovered to better select patients for treatment with drugs like bevacizumab.
- Immunotherapies will be developed to harness the immune system to fight lung cancer. Numerous vaccines are already in clinical development for lung cancer. There is proof of principle that drugs that enhance the immune system are effective in treating other solid tumors, such as melanoma.
- Oncogene blockade with tyrosine kinase inhibitors is effective therapy, but lung cancers quickly become resistant to this limited treatment strategy.
  - Combinations of oncogene blockade with upregulation of tumor suppressor genes or pro-apoptotic genes may enhance cancer kill.
  - New insights into cancer biochemistry will allow targeting of anaerobic glycolysis, which is a unique metabolic requirement of the most poorly differentiated cancer cells.
- Current chemotherapy drugs eliminate rapidly dividing cells. Cancer stem cells are impervious to these drugs. New discoveries will help to find and kill cancer stem cells, which will undoubtedly improve anticancer therapy and rates of cure.
- Technological advancements will allow for faster discovery of new cancer genes and targets.
  - The discovery of EGFR tyrosine kinase inhibitors from phase 1 study and establishing the EGFR mutant subgroup of NSCLC as an important new disease entitiy took 10 years. The discovery and successful targeting of ALK has only taken 4 years.
  - The first sequencing of the entire human genome was accomplished in 2000 with 15 years of work and billions of dollars of investment. Current technologies can sequence an entire human genome in a few weeks for less than $20,000.
  - The accelerated ability to sequence every gene in cancer DNA (the whole oncogenome) will undoubtedly

accelerate oncogene and tumor suppressor gene discovery as well as drug development.

■ As rates of cigarette smoking continue to decline in this country due to health-conscious tobacco policies, fewer patients will be at risk for lung cancer in this country than ever before.

* Unfortunately, smoking rates in China, Eastern Europe, and the Third World continue to rise.

* Combined with inferior healthcare systems to fight lung cancer, the global epidemic of lung cancer may increase even as we Americans enjoy our best triumphs in our fight against this deadliest of cancers.

Index

Note: Italicized page locators indicate photos/figures; tables are indicated with *t*.

Lightning Source UK Ltd.
Milton Keynes UK
UKOW030752191112

202409UK00002B/1/P